A PRIMER OF
BEHAVIORAL
PHARMACOLOGY

A PRIMER OF BEHAVIORAL PHARMACOLOGY

Concepts and Principles in the Behavioral Analysis of Drug Action

Peter L. Carlton

Department of Psychiatry UMDNJ—Rutgers Medical School Piscataway, New Jersey

W.H.Freeman and Company

New York   San Francisco

Library of Congress Cataloging in Publication Data

Carlton, Peter Lynn, 1931–
  A primer of behavioral pharmacology.
  Bibliography: p.
  Includes index.
  1. Psychopharmacology—Research. 2. Behavioral
assessment. I. Title. [DNLM: 1. Behavior—Drug effects.
2. Psychotropic drugs.   QV 77 C285p]
BF207.C28   1983   615'.78   83-9083

Printed in the United States of America

10 9 8 7 6 5 4 3 2 1

For Elizabeth

Contents

Acknowledgments

First and foremost, I want to express my gratitude to my wife, Janet Berson. Had it not been for her encouragement and patience there would have been, quite simply, no book.

I also want to thank John Falk and Leonard Hamilton for their criticisms of an earlier version of the manuscript. Their comments and suggestions vastly improved the present version.

Finally, I want to thank my secretary, Gail Kniffen. Her contributions were uniformly well beyond the call of duty.

Chapter 1
Introduction

THE PHYSIOLOGIC EFFECTS of drugs are truly remarkable. There are two basic reasons why this is so. First, drugs are extremely potent; a few thousandths of a gram of morphine, for example, will totally eliminate pain, and an equally small amount of an antibiotic can eradicate a disease. Second, drugs are extremely specific; morphine can eliminate pain but has no effect on the cause of disease, whereas the antibiotic can destroy a disease-causing organism without directly altering the perception of pain.

The effects of drugs on behavior are equally potent or specific, a fact that has been evident since humans first drank wine or smoked hashish. Yet the behavioral analysis of drug action has, compared to other aspects of pharmacology, only barely begun. Traditional pharmacology has understandably been focused on agents having demonstrable utility in the management of disease. Only relatively recently, however, have certain drugs been proved to have clinically useful effects on behavior.

The drug chlorpromazine, still used in the management of psychotic behavior, was the first widely-accepted agent shown to produce such beneficial effects. The introduction of chlorpromazine in 1954 began a new era in pharmacotherapy—one based solely on a medically relevant modification of behavior. More particularly, the effectiveness of chlorpromazine showed that the vastly disorganized behavior labeled psychotic can be controlled, at least in part, by certain drugs. The management of psychosis—deranged behavior—by such drugs is analogous to the control of the symptoms of diabetes—deranged metabolism—by insulin. Thus, as often happens, successful pharmacologic management of a disease set the occasion for a scientific turnabout (see Swazey and Reeds, 1978). In this case, both the disease and the management effected by the drug are behavioral. The results with chlorpromazine prompted recognition of *behavior* as a new facet of pharmacologic analysis.

We will return to this theme in Chapter 13 when we consider chlorpromazine and related drugs in detail. For the moment we will focus on chlorpromazine's direct impact on the field of behavioral pharmacology. We can get a sense of that impact by examining Figure 1–1: Behavioral pharmacology exploded from obscurity with the introduction of chlorpromazine; the field developed at a rapid rate in the period 1955–1963 and has continued to grow since that time.

This sudden development did not, however, occur in a vacuum. Indeed, two powerful forces converged to give it impetus. First, the behavioral effects of chlorpromazine prompted substantial government funding for research on the behavioral effects of drugs. At the same time, the pharmaceutical industry, recognizing that a new arena for sales was available to it, began to underwrite extensive research programs in behavioral pharmacology.

Yet another contributing factor was the powerful and sophisticated

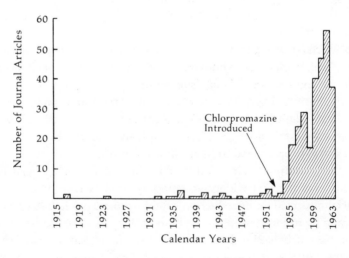

Figure 1–1. Numbers of publications in behavioral pharmacology for the period 1915–1963. (From Pickens, 1977)

behavioral technology that had independently developed within the field of psychology in the years following the publication of Skinner's *Behavior of Organisms* in 1938. This technology was ideally suited to the needs of the newly emergent discipline of behavioral pharmacology. Thus, there was an imminent research need and a way that the need could be met. A marriage of psychology and pharmacology was the result.

Unfortunately, the rapidity with which this union prospered also created a problem. Each scientific discipline has its own language, technology, and point of view. On the other hand, when a discipline matures very rapidly, those not privy to the discipline's inner workings can quickly find themselves outside looking in. Thus, there are many who recognize the importance of behavioral pharmacology but also find the research literature to be rather incomprehensible. This apparent obscurity is an artifact of the rapid development of the field, not an intrinsic characteristic of the discipline. The behavioral analysis of drug action is complex, and working through the details can sometimes be tedious, to be sure; but the subject is certainly not inaccessible, as we shall see in the chapters that lie ahead.

Our study of the behavioral analysis of drug action will focus on principles and conceptual problems in behavioral analysis, not on a mere listing of the behavioral effects of different drugs in different circumstances. We will not, therefore, be dealing with a compendium of established fact. However, the effects of a large variety of drugs will be used to illustrate particular conceptual issues. Thus, by Chapter 17, we will have developed a general, but not detailed, picture of the behavioral effects of most drugs of current interest.[1]

Another aspect of our study of behavioral pharmacology is an emphasis on a specific technology. This emphasis on so-called "operant" procedures certainly does not mean that they are necessarily the ultimate concern of behavioral pharmacology; it does mean that these procedures have a demonstrated analytic power that has, in turn, led to their virtually universal adoption within the discipline. We must understand this technology if we are to understand the subject itself.

The behavioral techniques we will be considering are not simple; more to the point, the data that they generate are not simple. As we shall see, the behavioral effects of drugs can be vastly complicated because they are determined by a wide range of variables in addition to the drug itself. The popularly held view that each drug has a single behavioral action that is universally realized is an utterly wrong idea.

Our ultimate problem, then, will be to develop ways in which a degree of order can be brought to this enormously complex field. We will begin to tackle this problem by examining the ways in which the behavioral effects of drugs can be measured. This is the topic of Section I.

NOTE

1. Because the general features of the actions of different drugs are emphasized, secondary literature sources are usually given. Thus, many unquestionably important individual studies of particular problems have not been cited; most of them can, however, be found in the secondary sources. (Materials that appeared after the early months of 1982 have not been included.)

Section 1
The Measurement of Drug Effect

IF WE ARE to undertake a behavioral analysis of drug action, we must, of course, administer a drug and measure some behavior. Unfortunately, the undertaking is not as simple as this.

In the first place, there are many ways in which behavior can be measured; we will examine a variety of these ways in Chapter 2. More to the point, different behaviors are differentially sensitive to drug action. That is, no one drug has a uniform effect on all behaviors.

We will begin to explore that note of complexity as we move into Chapter 3. In addition, we will encounter yet another kind of complexity: Characterization of drug action hinges not only on the drug chosen for study but, just as important, on the amount administered. Although this point seems self-evident, the fact remains that the research literature is replete with attempts to characterize behavioral effect on the basis of a single dose of drug. As we shall see, attempts of this kind make no sense whatsoever.

In Chapter 4, we will begin to put together some of this information. We will focus on two issues: one that is specific to the measurement process itself and one that is more generally relevant to behavioral analysis. The specific issue concerns the way in which a single characteristic of different behaviors—their rate—can determine the drug effect measured. The more general issue, derived from this concept, amounts to the following: We cannot think of the behavioral changes induced by drugs in terms of simple input–output relationships ("drug in–behavior out"); rather, we must think of these changes as occurring within a complex system of which drug action is only one part. We will repeatedly return to this theme as we proceed.

Chapter 2
Basic Behavioral Procedures

IN THIS CHAPTER we will focus on descriptions of those behavioral procedures that have become so pervasive that they can be regarded as fundamental to behavioral pharmacology. Particular procedures designed for particular problems are not included in the following discussion unless they have also been shown to be generally useful. However, even though only a limited number of procedures are considered, some readers may find the material a trifle overwhelming; accordingly, these procedures are summarized in a review section that follows their initial presentation.

In one sense, the material covered merely introduces a very elementary language in which different terms refer to different ways in which behavior can be engendered and measured; behavioral pharmacology, like any other scientific discipline, has its own language—one that must be mastered if it is to be understood.

SHOCK-CONTROLLED BEHAVIOR

We first consider a category of procedures that involves the use of electric shock to control behavior. These procedures are discriminated avoidance, nondiscriminated avoidance, punishment, "go–no go" avoidance, and the conditioned emotional response.

DISCRIMINATED AVOIDANCE

The discriminated avoidance procedure in its rudimentary form is simplicity itself. A stimulus such as a light or a buzzer is presented; a short time thereafter electric shock is turned on. The animal confronts these two events while in some sort of apparatus that allows for, first, contact with the shock and, second, a way to get away from it. Thus, a rat, for example, might be placed in a chamber having a floor made up of metal bars that permit the shock to be delivered to the animal's feet; it might be able to get away from the shock by running to a part of the floor that is not electrified, or by pressing a lever that turns off the shock, or by jumping onto a small shelf above the floor. When the animal responds in one of these ways, or whatever other way provided in the experiment, the animal is said to have **escaped.** Recall, however, that the shock is also announced by a signal (e.g., a tone) that precedes it. Thus, the animal has the opportunity to **avoid** the impending shock by emitting the prescribed behavior before the shock actually occurs.[1]

The discriminated avoidance procedure has two general forms called "one-way" and "two-way."

One-way Avoidance   Imagine a box that has the relative dimensions of a shoe box but is about three times as large. The box is divided into two equal compartments by a small barrier over which a rat can easily jump. In addition, the floor of the box is made up of grids in both compartments; these two compartments can be independently electrified. Suppose that the animal is in the left-hand compartment when the warning signal comes on, and that electric shock will be applied to the floor on the left side in 30 seconds. If the rat jumps the barrier into the right-hand compartment within the 30 seconds, it avoids the shock. If it fails to do so, however, it can escape the shock that has been turned on by then jumping into the right-hand compartment. (Most rats learn to avoid the impending shock in a very few exposures to the signal–shock contingency.) If the animal is always placed in the left-hand compartment prior to the initiation of the signal shock trial, then the avoidance or escape response is "one-way" in the sense that the rat always moves from left to right.

Two-way Avoidance   Consider the oversized shoe box again. The animal may not be removed from the box after the trial; rather, it may be allowed to remain in the right-hand compartment until the next sig-

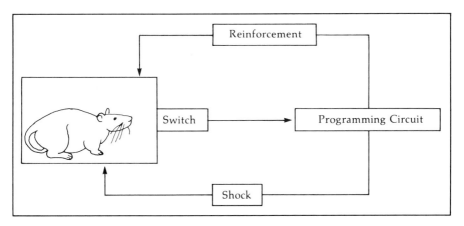

Figure 2–1. Schematic of response chamber used to study behavior maintained by various contingencies. (Modified from Pickens, 1977)

nal–shock presentation. In this case, the animal will be required to move from right to left after it has previously moved from left to right. Thus, the animal will be required to shuttle between the two compartments—a "two-way" response.[2],[3]

NONDISCRIMINATED AVOIDANCE

Although nondiscriminated avoidance is sometimes called "Sidman avoidance" (in recognition of Murray Sidman, its inventor), we will use the more descriptive "nondiscriminated" because this term explains the essence of the procedure: There is an avoidance contingency, but the impending shock is unsignaled by an exteroceptive stimulus. This does not mean that the shock is literally nondiscriminated, because, as we shall see, animals do come to discriminate the fact that shock is about to be delivered; what it does mean is that there is no scheduled external warning signal, as there is in the case of discriminated avoidance.

Suppose an animal is placed in a chamber like that crudely schematized in Figure 2–1. (The figure also depicts a device for delivering reinforcements to the animal; the use of this device will be discussed shortly.) Electric shock can be delivered to the rat via the grid floor on which it stands. This shock is controlled in two ways: The experimenter can control it by way of programming circuitry, or the animal can control it by depressing the lever in the chamber and thereby closing a switch. In effect, the animal has a means of interacting with the program to determine shock delivery.

The key to this program is a clock; the animal can interact with the program because its responses (lever depressions) close a switch that resets the clock. Suppose, for example, that the clock is set for 30 seconds. When that time has run out, the clock delivers a shock to the grid floor. But the clock can be reset to zero by the animal's response so that delivery of shock need never occur. The following sequence illustrates the point: Clock starts, 10 seconds elapse, rat responds; clock resets and starts again, 25 seconds elapse, rat again responds; clock resets and starts again; and so on. Thus, by responding at least once every 30 seconds, the rat can avoid all shocks.

Of course, with an untrained rat, the clock does run out and shock is delivered in one of two ways. In one version of the procedure, a single shock is delivered for a brief period (one-half second, say) over which the animal has no control. The clock then starts over again. In other versions, the animal receives a series of brief inescapable shocks (every second, for example) until it does respond.

The interval set on the clock just discussed is termed the **response–shock (RS) interval** because it is the time that must elapse between a response (and the consequent resetting and restarting of the clock) and the next shock (30 seconds in the example). In the case where repeated brief, inescapable shocks are used, the interval between such shocks may be separately programmed; this interval is called the **shock–shock (SS) interval.**

Now suppose that the RS interval is set at 20 seconds (RS20) and the SS interval is set at 3 seconds (SS3). Further suppose that the rat has had extensive training: It responds 10 seconds after its previous response, then 5 seconds thereafter, and then again 19 seconds thereafter; it then does not respond within 20 seconds. A brief shock is delivered at that time and every three seconds thereafter until the animal does respond. This response stops the SS interval and again starts the RS interval. In this case, responses emitted during the SS periods are the analog of escape responses in discriminated avoidance.

As a final illustration, suppose the rat makes the three responses at the intervals described above (i.e., 10, 5, and 19 seconds followed by

Table 2–1

Event	R	R	R	S	S	S	R	R
Interevent interval (sec)	10	5	19	20	3	3	2	15
Elapsed time (sec)	10	15	34	54	57	60	62	77
Cumulated responses		1	2	3				4	5

the 20 seconds without a response). At that time a shock is delivered. Now suppose that the animal takes two more shocks, responds 2 seconds after the last shock, and again responds 15 seconds later. This sequence of five responses takes 77 seconds and follows the pattern shown in Table 2–1 (R denotes a response; S, shock delivery).

Once an animal has been trained with this technique, it comes to emit responses at a low, very stable rate that is attuned to the magnitude of the RS interval; the shorter the RS interval, the more rapidly the animal will respond. This rate will be essentially invariant over the course of several hours.

PUNISHMENT PROCEDURES

In punishment procedures the animal is given an electric shock if it emits some prescribed response. In everyday parlance, the animal has been punished and, as a result, stops making the response. (Recall that we first considered this effect in the context of two-way avoidance; see Note 2.)

Punishment of Reinforced Behavior   For study of the effects of punishment, the response to be punished must, of course, be emitted in the first place. An obvious way to arrange for this is first to train the animal to emit some response and then, once it is regularly doing so, to punish that response and thereby produce a **suppression** of the previously trained behavior. A widely used version of this technique involves training animals to press a lever in a chamber like that shown in Figure 2–1. For example, a food-deprived rat can be given reinforcement (for pressing the lever) by the small food pellets that are delivered into the chamber. (Reinforcement procedures will be discussed more fully in the section "Reinforced Behavior" later in this chapter.) Because of the reinforcement, the animal will repeatedly press the lever. The procedure can be so arranged that a stimulus (e.g., a tone) is presented and that responses during the stimulus will result in the delivery of reinforcement *and* in a brief electric shock to the grid floor of the chamber. Thus, responses are punished if they are emitted during the stimulus.

Under these circumstances the animal comes to stop responding during the stimulus but to continue to respond when the stimulus is absent. Thus, the technique provides a way of determining the effect of a drug on the general ability of the animal to respond (when the stimulus is not on) as well as any effect that the drug may have on the behavior that has been suppressed by the shock (when the stimulus is on).

There have been a number of variations of this procedure, including simpler versions. For example, a water-deprived rat is allowed to drink water; it is also shocked in the act of drinking. Thus, a high level of responding (drinking) can be easily engendered and its suppression by punishment simply recorded.

Punishment of Exploratory Behavior   A second general type of punishment technique, one that does not include reinforcement of the to-be-punished behavior, involves exploration of a novel environment. The following example illustrates the character of the procedure. Suppose our rat is put into a chamber that contains not a lever to be depressed but a small shelf onto which the animal can jump. When placed on the shelf the rat will step down onto the grid floor of the box to explore its environment. But if the grid floor is electrified, exploration will be abruptly suppressed. The animal will spend virtually all of its time on the shelf, whereas it would spend relatively little time there were the punishment contingency not in effect.

There have been a number of variants on this technique as well, each involving the variations in response that is suppressed, but the essence of them all is to be found in the procedure just described.

"GO–NO GO" AVOIDANCE

Other, more complex experimental techniques have been devised to produce correspondingly more complicated behavior. For example, a punishment contingency can be added to an avoidance contingency to produce *"go–no go" avoidance.*

The "go" means that, in the presence of one stimulus, the animal can avoid shock only if it moves to a second compartment of the chamber, just as is the case in discriminated avoidance situations. The "no go" is the part that adds the complexity: In the presence of another stimulus, the animal must *not* move into the second compartment if it is to avoid shock. If it does so, shock will be delivered just as in a punishment situation. The aim here is to build into a single animal two different behaviors, each related to a separate procedure. Whether or not there is much gain is, however, an open question; the "go–no go" arrangement does allow direct and simultaneous comparisons of the effects of drug on two behaviors, but the behaviors themselves may be riddled with complex interactions. That is, it is unlikely that "go" behavior is the same as behavior generated in a discriminated avoidance procedure without a "no go" contingency. Conversely, it is unlikely that the "no go" behavior is functionally the same as punished behavior in the absence of the "go."

THE CONDITIONED EMOTIONAL RESPONSE

The final technique that involves electric shock is called the conditioned emotional response (CER). For this technique, an animal is again placed in a chamber that contains a lever that it can depress. Such responses are reinforced, as they are in punishment procedures. As is also the case in punishment procedures, a signal is presented to indicate that a shock contingency is in effect. The presence of that signal indicates that a brief, inescapable electric shock is forthcoming. It is the inevitability of that shock that distinguishes the CER technique from punishment procedures: In punishment procedures, no shocks are delivered if the animal fails to respond. In CER, the shock is delivered independently of the rat's behavior.

As it happens, the lever pressing of the animal is suppressed when the signal is presented, just as it is in the punishment situation. In CER, the animal presses the lever at some regular rate but stops responding when the signal is present. This signal indicates that, after some prescribed time, a shock will inevitably be delivered. In the case of a punishment technique, the animal is also responding at some rate in the absence of the signal, stops responding in the presence of that signal, and by doing so, does not receive shock. The procedural differences between the two are small. In one case, the animal can eliminate the potential of shock by failing to respond; in the second case, the animal cannot do so because the shock is delivered regardless of the behavior emitted during the signal.

IMPLICATIONS OF DIFFERENCES AMONG PROCEDURES

In general, the different procedures involving electric shock provide three kinds of behavioral indices for measuring drug effect: avoidance, escape, and suppression. If there are only three basic indices, however, why are there actually seven different techniques in general use?

A part of the answer lies in the dictates of a particular experiment. A certain experimental question might, for example, be better answered if external stimuli were not involved. Thus, nondiscriminated avoidance rather than discriminated avoidance might be better suited to the problem.

A second and much more cogent part of the answer lies in the subtle differences that seemingly very similar procedures introduce. These differences generate, in turn, different sensitivities to drug action. As we shall see in Chapter 16, for example, the actions of certain drugs are much more reliably detected by discriminated avoidance procedures than by nondiscriminated avoidance procedures. Similarly, punishment procedures are more useful in detecting the actions of certain drugs than is CER. That is, despite the superficial similarity of the two—both induce a suppression of ongoing behavior—they are not identical in their sensitivity to drug action. We will consider these differences in Chapter 15. For the moment we can focus on the more general point: Differences in procedure that are apparently very small can produce profound effects on the behavioral changes produced by drugs.

REINFORCED BEHAVIOR

In procedures involving reinforced behavior, the animal is placed in a chamber with a lever available to it. A rat (or monkey) can depress the lever with its forepaws and thereby close a switch connected to programming equipment located outside the chamber (as in Figure 2–1). For a pigeon, a small disc rather than a lever is mounted on the wall of the box; the bird can peck at this disc and thereby close the switch.

A deprived animal can be trained to emit these responses to lever or disc by the delivery of a small amount of food or water into the box following each response. (The small amounts of food or water are made available by means of the reinforcement device schematized in Figure 2–1). Alternatively, as is most commonly the case, responses are only intermittently reinforced according to some programmed schedule.

VARIABLE RATIO SCHEDULE

One of the simplest of such programmed schedules is called *variable ratio* (VR). In the everyday world, the VR schedule is a part of the programming that goes into a slot machine: Each time the lever on a slot machine is pulled, there is a chance of a payoff; the payoff, if it occurs, may be any of various amounts of money. The VR used in experimentation refers only to the first contingency: Not every response will pay off—but some will.

The *schedule* determines the relationship of responding to reinforcement; there may be a payoff after 10 responses, then after only 1 response, again after 23 responses, and so on. (The aspect of a variable amount for each reinforcement, as in a slot machine, is not a part of the arrangement.)

The VR schedule is characterized by the average number of responses required of the animal for a reinforcement to be delivered. Thus, *VR20* would indicate that reinforcements might be delivered after 5, 52, 12, 3, and 28 responses; the sum of the required responses is 100: the average is $100/5 = 20$. (In practice, VR schedules are much more complex and variable with respect to the actual values that enter into the average.) The phrase "variable ratio" thus summarizes the fact that there is a ratio of responses to reinforcements; this relationship is not constant and can, therefore, be expressed only as an average.

Such schedules generate extremely high, stable rates of responding. Again consider the behavior generated at the slot machine: Responding goes on and on despite the known fact that continued responding may result in a net loss; casinos are not, after all, charitable organizations.

FIXED RATIO SCHEDULE

Just as reinforcements can be scheduled to be delivered after variable numbers of responses have been emitted, they can also be scheduled for delivery after a fixed number of responses. This arrangement is called *fixed ratio* (FR) and is characterized by the number of responses required for each reinforcement. Thus, *FR20* would mean that the animal be delivered a reinforcement after 20 responses, again after the next 20, and so on. A "real life" analog of this schedule is a "piece rate"; the worker is paid for each piece of work performed, although each such "piece" may require a number of responses. For example, an employee at an egg-packing facility who earns a set amount for each carton packed is paid on a FR12 schedule.

FR schedules generate high and stable rates of responding, just as VR schedules do. However, FR has a second characteristic that appears in the animal's behavior when the value of the ratio is sufficiently high. Although this value will vary substantially with different species of animal, animals show a pause in responding after the delivery of reinforcement at some value of the FR. A rat, for example, may emit 50 responses at a very high rate, typically without any substantial interruption whatsoever. When it receives its reinforcement, however, it will not begin responding again for a notable period of time. After this period of pausing has elapsed, responding at the typical high rate will again be resumed until another 50 responses have been emitted and the next reinforcement has been received. There will then be another pause, and so on. With smaller ratios, the duration of the pauses will be shorter.

These pauses are not simply a result of fatigue, as might at first be supposed. We know this because an animal working on a VR50, say, will not show such pausing. In VR50, the overall response requirements are the same as those in FR50. It thus appears that the critical difference in the behaviors inheres in the fixed relation of reinforcement to response requirement. In FR, a subsequent reinforcement will never occur until an additional 50 responses are emitted, whereas there is no such certainty in VR. That is, it appears that the delivery of reinforcement in FR itself comes to signal the *un*availability of reinforcement and, thus, comes to control a post-reinforcement pause in responding.

VARIABLE INTERVAL SCHEDULE

It is also possible to schedule reinforcements so that they are available after irregular intervals of time. This schedule, called *variable interval* (VI), is characterized by the average of the intervals between reinforcement availability. Thus, in VI2, reinforcement might be available 115 seconds after the last reinforcement, again 24 seconds later, then 186 seconds later, then 231 and finally 44 seconds later. The total time is 600 seconds (115 + 24 + 186 + 231 + 44); 600/5 reinforcements = 120 seconds per reinforcement = 2 minutes; hence, VI2.

The key word in the definition above is "availability." A VI schedule is arranged so that a reinforcement can be claimed after a given interval, but it can be claimed only if the animal responds. An animal can, therefore, lose time in the sense that the longer it fails to respond once a reinforcement has been made available, the greater will be the interval before the next reinforcement is made available.

Animals do adjust to this feature of the schedule and, because reinforcement availability is unpredictable, come to respond at essentially invariant, stable rates that are accommodated to the particular VI. A VI2, for example, will control a rate higher than that with a VI3. Furthermore, because a very few reinforcements will sustain the desired behavior, it is possible to obtain rates of responding that are maintained over very protracted periods. That is, response rate does not wane because of the waning of motivation that would occur with an accumulation of reinforcements delivered at short intervals.

FIXED INTERVAL SCHEDULE

When reinforcements for responding are made available at regular intervals, the behavior generated differs markedly from that seen with VI (relatively low, very stable rates), with VR (very high, stable rates), or with FR (high, stable rates often characterized by pauses in responding after reinforcement). With a *fixed interval* schedule (FI), the animal typically pauses after each reinforcement and gradually increases its rate of responding as the interval runs out.

If reinforcements are made available once every 2 minutes (again, "available" but not delivered until a response occurs), the schedule is noted as *FI2*. The trained rat working on this schedule typically does not respond for several seconds after reinforcement and then emits a few responses, then a few more at a higher rate, and so on, until a high terminal rate is reached just prior to reinforcement availability. Thus, FI is like FR in that it generates post-reinforcement pauses but differs from FR in that there is a gradual rate change rather than the abrupt shift to the high terminal rate of FR.

DIFFERENTIAL REINFORCEMENT OF LOW RATES OF RESPONDING (DRL)

The letters *DRL* denote a schedule that differentially (*D*) reinforces (*R*) low (*L*) rates of responding. The DRL schedule has a kinship with non-discriminated avoidance in that both depend on a clock that is reset by the animal's responses. In nondiscriminated avoidance, the clock delivers shock if the animal fails to respond and thereby to reset it during the RS interval. In DRL, the clock makes a reinforcement available when it runs down, and as in the avoidance contingency, it will do so only if the animal has not responded. Thus, in avoidance, failure to respond eventuates in shock delivery, whereas in DRL, failure to respond sets the occasion for reinforcement of a subsequent response.

The notation *DRL20* indicates that the animal is required to delay its responses—to fail to respond—for at least 20 seconds and *then* to respond to claim the reinforcement made available by the passage of the prescribed time. Animals require extensive training on this schedule before they develop stable response patterns. The final performance is, as we would suppose, a very low, steady rate of response attuned to the interresponse time demanded; for example, DRL40 would generate rates lower than those seen with DRL20.

REVIEW OF BEHAVIORAL PROCEDURES

The basic procedures involving electric shock are schematically summarized in Figures 2–2 and 2–3.

Discriminated avoidance is described in the upper portion of Figure 2–2. Note that, with the passage of time (the top row), the signal (shown

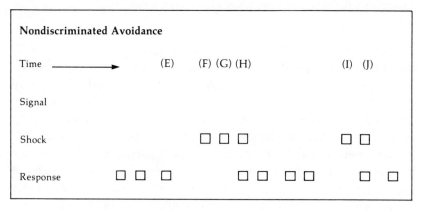

Figure 2–2. Schematic description of discriminated (top) and nondiscriminated (bottom) avoidance procedures.

in the second row) is presented at regular intervals following each response (the bottom row); failure to respond rapidly enough results in shock delivery (the third row), and termination of both shock and signal is contingent on response emission (an escape response, at *A*). Responses that occur early in the signal period terminate the signal and eliminate the scheduled shock (avoidance responses, as at *B* and *C;* note that the response at *C* occurs more rapidly than at *B*). Another instance of a failure to avoid followed by an escape is shown at *D*. A nondiscriminated avoidance schedule is schematized in the lower portion of Figure 2–2. There are, of course, no signal presentations, but shocks can be avoided by responses that are emitted at intervals less than the RS interval (the time between *E* and *F*). A failure to respond within this

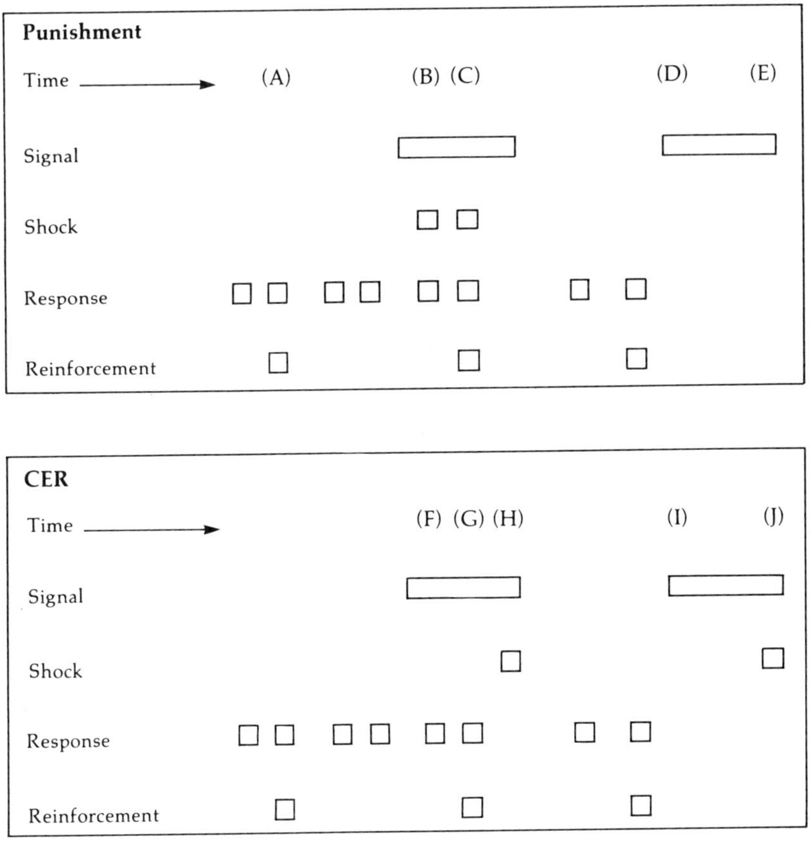

Figure 2–3. Schematic description of punishment (top) and CER (bottom) procedures.

interval (at F) eventuates in a shock delivery that is repeated in the absence of a response; the time between F and G and between G and H is the SS interval. Response emission (as at H) reinstates the RS interval. Following a sequence of responses, failure to respond within the RS interval (at I) again results in shock delivery and initiates another SS interval; in this instance, we see that the SS interval is terminated by the response at J.

Punishment and CER procedures are summarized in Figure 2–3. The sequence of events shown in the upper portion describes a hypothetical punishment procedure. Responses in the absence of a signal (as at A) are intermittently reinforced (as on a VI schedule), whereas responses during the signal may be reinforced but also eventuate in shock delivery (both reinforcement and shock occur at C, but only shock occurs at B). A second signal presentation (at D) completely suppresses responding in that no responses are emitted.

The sequence of responding and reinforcement in the CER procedure shown in the lower portion of Figure 2–3 is identical to that in the punishment sequence. This arbitrary arrangement highlights the salient difference between punishment and CER procedures: The responses at F and G do not produce shock (in contrast to B and C), but shock does occur at H, independently of response emission. Thus, shock is response-contingent in the case of punishment but response-independent in the case of CER. This difference is further emphasized by the comparison between D–E and I–J. In the former case, no responses occur during the signal (D–E), and no shocks are delivered; in the CER procedure, however, shock does occur (at J) even though no responses are emitted during the signal (I–J).

The relevant features of the reinforcement schedules discussed are diagrammed in Figures 2–4 and 2–5; the two ratio schedules (VR and FR) are schematized in Figure 2–4, and time-based schedules are shown in Figure 2–5.

The sequence of responses shown in the upper portion of Figure 2–4 results in reinforcement availability on three occasions (A, C, and E). Note that different numbers of responses (2, 3, and 1) provide for this availability but that the reinforcements themselves are not delivered until the subsequent response is emitted in each case. Thus, reinforcements occur (at B, D, and F) after different numbers of responses have been emitted (3, 4, and 2). There is, then, a variable relationship between responses and reinforcements. In this case, 9 responses produce 3 reinforcements; the schedule is therefore VR3.

A different relationship of response to reinforcement is characteristic of FR (the lower portion of Figure 2–4). In this case, reinforcements are made available after a fixed number of responses (4 responses as at G and I) but delivered only after the emission of an additional response (at H and J). Thus, the schedule requires a total of 10 responses for the delivery of 2 reinforcements; the schedule is FR5.

A variable interval schedule is schematized at the top of Figure 2–5. Note that the intervals between reinforcement delivery (at B, D, and F) and subsequent availability (at C and E) are variable; also note that these reinforcements can be claimed by response emission only during periods of reinforcement availability. If the entire period shown is 3 minutes, the schedule is VI1 (3 reinforcements/3 minutes).

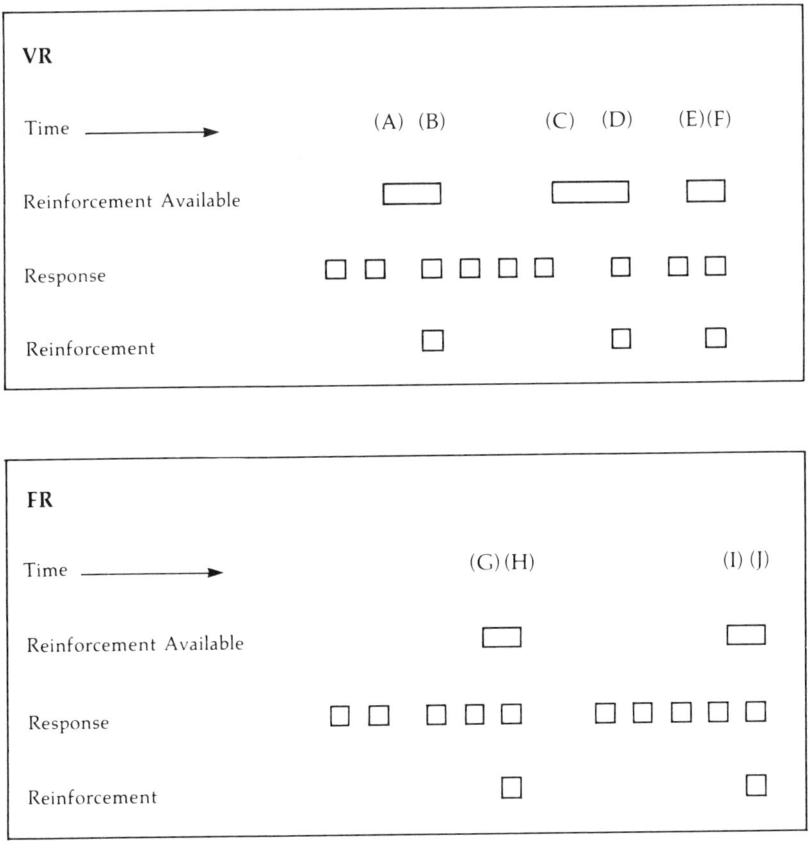

Figure 2–4. Schematic description of VR (top) and FR (bottom) schedules of reinforcement.

This arrangement is to be contrasted with that for FI, schematized in the middle panel of Figure 2–5. Although reinforcement availability is independent of response emission, as in VI, there is, with FI, a fixed, temporal interval between reinforcement delivery and subsequent availability; the interval G–H equals I–J in contrast to B–C *versus* D–E in the illustration for VI. Also note that there is a greater likelihood of response emission as these intervals run out (i.e., there is a tendency for a post-reinforcement pause in responding to occur after G and, especially, after I). If the entire period shown is 3 minutes, the schedule is FI1.

The relation of responding to reinforcement for a DRL schedule is illustrated in the bottom panel of Figure 2–5. In this schedule, reinforce-

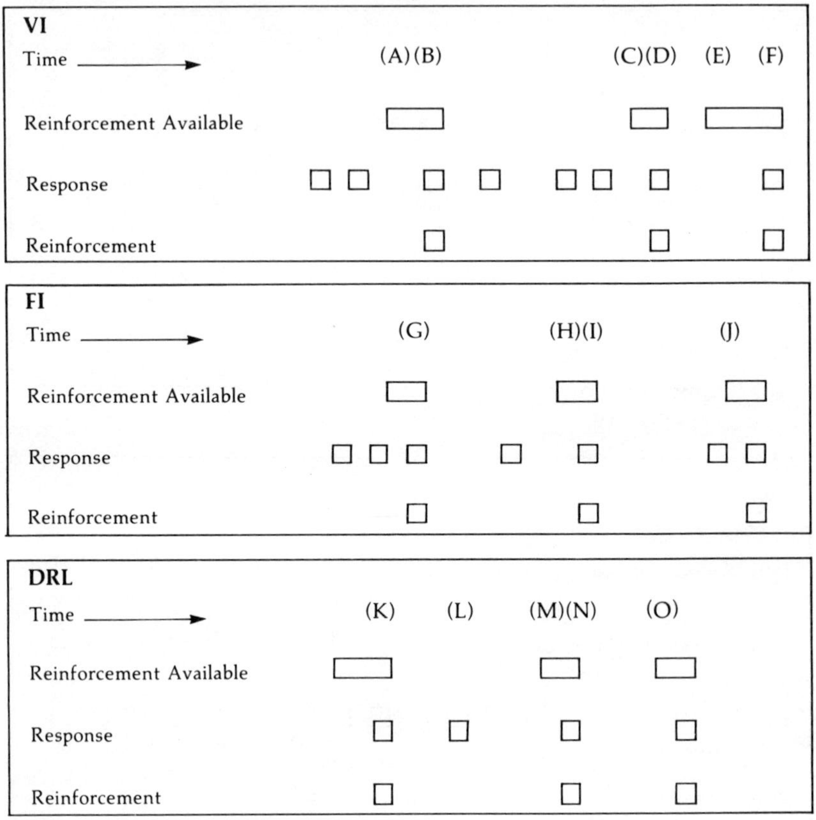

Figure 2–5. Schematic description of VI (top), FI (middle), and DRL (bottom) reinforcement schedules.

ments are not available until the animal has failed to respond for a fixed period of time. Thus, reinforcement delivery (at K) initiates an interval that is interrupted by a response (at L); the interval is then reinitiated (also at L) only to be completed (at M) because of the absence of responding in the $L–M$ interval. When the reinforcement thus made available is claimed (at N), a new interval is initiated and completed without interruption. Low rates of responding, therefore, increase reinforcement availability (the $N–O$ interval is shorter than $K–M$), but a response is required if the animal is to capitalize on this availability. (If the $L–M$ and $N–O$ intervals each are 20 seconds, the schedule is DRL20; recall that DRL schedules are denoted in seconds, not minutes as with VI and FI.)

CUMULATIVE RECORDS OF RESPONDING

Each of the schedules of reinforcement previously discussed generates a different pattern of responding. Let us now consider the characteristics of these patterns.[4]

The responses that an animal emits can be recorded in a variety of ways: the total number emitted in an experimental session, the number emitted in the successive periods that make up the session (e.g., total responses per 10-minute period), and so on. Tabulations of these kinds do not, of course, provide a continuous record of the moment-to-moment occurrence of responses. However, such a continuous record can be generated by allowing an animal to "draw" its own record with the aid of a device called a *cumulative recorder*, which adds the responses as they occur over time. A schematic version of such a recorder is shown in Figure 2–6. Because each response by the animal closes a switch, it is possible to arrange a circuit so that each response activates the electrically operated pen, which in turn moves one step upward with each response.

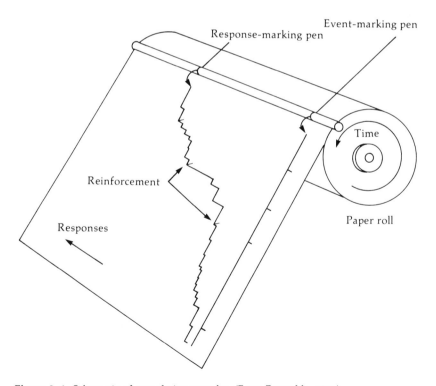

Figure 2–6. Schematic of cumulative recorder. (From Reynolds, 1968)

Suppose that an animal emits the sequence of 10 responses shown across the top of the upper graph in Figure 2–7. (Each upward deflection indicates a single response.) Further suppose that the eighth response is reinforced. This sequence, when cumulated, would generate the record shown in the middle of the figure. (Note that reinforcement is indicated by a diagonal hash mark on the cumulative record.)

Typical experimental procedures involve a multitude of responses

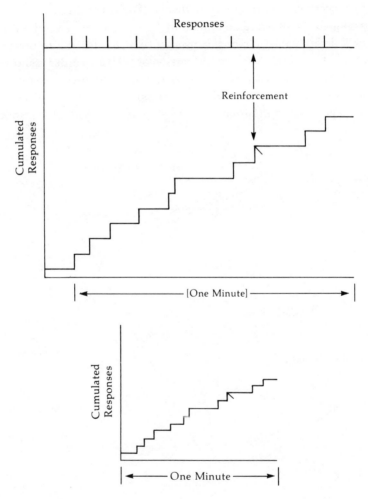

Figure 2–7. Responses are emitted (top) and cumulated (middle and bottom). The cumulative record shown at the bottom is a one-half reduction of the middle record.

and may extend for hours rather than for the 1 minute shown in Figure 2–7. It is, therefore, necessary to reduce the scale of the record to accommodate the hundreds of responses that may be emitted in the course of several hours. The record shown at the bottom of the figure is a one-half reduction of the cumalative record above it. Further reductions would obliterate the "steps" so that the record appears to be a continuous line (see Figure 2–8).

Even without the "steps" indicating individual responses, a cumulative record may show distinct angles composed of horizontal and nonhorizontal lines, as in Figure 2–8. Horizontal portions of the record indicate periods during which *no responses* occur. In Figure 2–8, the record shows that there are marked pauses after each reinforcement (the diagonal hash marks). According to the scale given at the lower right, pauses vary from about a minute (at *a*) to more than 10 minutes (at *b*).

The nonhorizontal portions—slopes—of such cumulative records indicate *rates of response.* In Figure 2–8, representative rates for the particular cumulative recorder used are given in the scale; the animal either is not responding (horizontal portions post-reinforcement) or is responding at a very high rate (nearly vertical slope, about 3 responses per second).

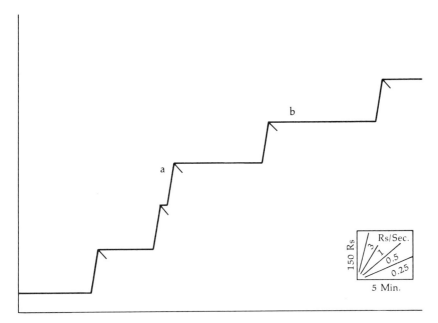

Figure 2–8. Sample cumulative record for an animal (a pigeon) that had been given extensive training on FR 120. (From Ferster and Skinner, 1957)

This pattern of responding is, as noted earlier, characteristic of FR at high ratios. The patterns typical of FR and other schedules previously discussed are shown in the schematic cumulative records in Figure 2–9. A summary of the characteristic features for each type of schedule follows:

1. VI: Intermittent reinforcements (the diagonal hash marks on the records) and steady rates attuned to the average VI (the value of the VI in *A* is less than in *B*)
2. FI: Reinforcements available at fixed intervals, a gradual increase in rate during each interval with overall rate attuned to the FI (the FI in *A* is less than in *B*)

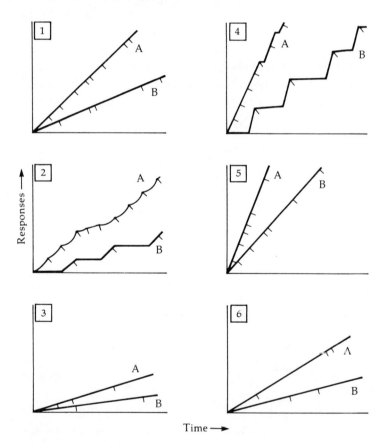

Figure 2–9. Sample cumulative records of responding maintained by different schedules of reinforcement. The schedules are VI *(1)*, FI *(2)*, DRL *(3)*, FR *(4)*, VR *(5)*, and nondiscriminated avoidance *(6)*.

3. DRL: Reinforcements available only after a fixed period of no re-sponding and low rates attuned to the value of the DRL (*A* less than *B*)

4. FR: Reinforcements available after a fixed number of responses and high rates with post-reinforcement pauses increasing with greater FR values (*A* is less than *B*)

5. VR: Reinforcements available after variable numbers of responses and relatively high rates attuned to the average VR (the VR in *A* is less than in *B*)

6. Nondiscriminated avoidance: Analogous to DRL in that shocks (the diagonal hash marks) are delivered after a fixed period of no re-sponding and rates are attuned to the RS interval (less in *A* than in *B*)

The behaviors controlled by such schedules can be studied in isolation or combined in a variety of ways. We shall briefly consider such combinations in the following section.

COMPLEX SCHEDULES AND THEIR INTERACTION

The schedules of reinforcement that we have considered can be combined so that different patterns of behavior can be studied within a single animal. A variety of such complex schedules has been employed (for a detailed discussion, see Ferster and Skinner, 1957); for purposes of illustration we will consider the most widely used of all complex schedules, the multiple schedule.

MULTIPLE SCHEDULES

A multiple schedule (*Mult*) typically incorporates two of the simpler schedules already discussed. When one schedule is in effect, one stimulus (e.g., a light) is turned on; when another schedule is in effect, another stimulus (e.g., a tone) is on. Under these conditions and with sufficient training, animals come to respond to each of the schedules in a way that is characteristic of the behavior generated by the schedules in isolation. If, for example, FR is scheduled when one stimulus is presented (e.g., a blue light) and VI is presented during a second stimulus (e.g., a red light), the behaviors characteristic of each schedule will appear—that is, high rates with pausing after reinforcement during the FR component (blue light on) and low, stable rates during the VI component (red light on). This schedule is noted as *Mult*FRVI.

SCHEDULE INTERACTIONS

Although the patterns of responding are characteristic of the schedules in isolation, these behaviors are not necessarily responsive to experimental manipulations in the same way that they would be if only one schedule were in effect. For example, because an animal comes to behave in a way characteristic of FR in one stimulus and in a way characteristic of VI in another, it does not necessarily follow that these behaviors are functionally identical to those that occur in isolation (FR without a VI component, or VI without FR). That is, the schedules may interact.

The following example, involving a well-known drug—alcohol (ethanol), illustrates the kinds of interaction that can occur. In a study by Barrett and Stanley (1980), animals were first trained on a two-component multiple schedule; one component was FI and the other was FR (the schedule of reinforcement was thus *Mult*FIFR). The value of the FI was held constant at 3 minutes, but the FR requirement was varied, ranging from 30 to 150 responses per reinforcement. The effects of different doses of ethanol were evaluated at each FR value, but the other schedule was maintained at FI3.

Barrett and Stanley found that, under control conditions, overall levels of FI responding were essentially constant regardless of the FR requirement in the other component. Despite this relative invariance in FI responding under control conditions, however, the effects of ethanol on FI responding *did* vary as a function of the FR, as illustrated in Figure 2–10. The plotted values in the figure are percentages of control. Thus, values above the horizontal dashed line indicate that ethanol increased responding; whereas values below it indicate a decrease relative to control.

Recall that our primary concern here is responding in the FI component and that the value of the FI was constant throughout the experiment. As Figure 2–10 shows, however, this constancy of FI did not produce a constancy of drug effect. Clearly, the schedule in the other component of the multiple schedule changed the character of the drug effect. In particular, when the opposite component was FR60, the effect of ethanol on FI responding was generally decremental at all doses; when the opposite component was FR150, ethanol actually increased responding at the intermediate doses and was relatively less effective in decreasing FI responding at the highest dose.

This single example illustrates a particularly important general point: Variations in procedure can profoundly alter the effect of a drug. We

FI Responding

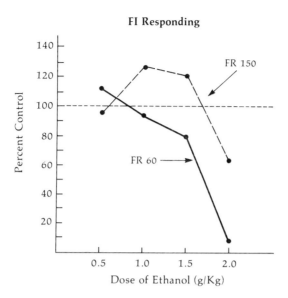

Figure 2–10. Variation in the effects of ethanol on FI responding due to differences in the FR component of a *Mult* FRFI schedule. The value of the FI was held constant at 3 minutes, but the FR component was either 60 or 150. (Redrawn from Barret and Stanley, 1980)

might assume, for example, that the behaviors studied by Barrett and Stanley are independent of each other (i.e., that the FR responding is the same as that which occurs in the absence of a FI schedule and that the FI behavior is the same as that which occurs in the absence of an FR schedule). In fact, this assumption appears to be supported by the observation that FI responding is essentially unchanged by variations in the FR requirement under control conditions. FI behavior thus appears to be independent of the FR schedule. With the introduction of a drug, however, we find that the assumption of independence is utterly wrong—the effect of ethanol (as seen in the FI component) is very much a function of the "context" (the FR requirement) in which it occurs. Related considerations are pertinent to some of the issues discussed in the following section.

GENERAL USE OF TECHNIQUES

The procedures discussed in this chapter are those that have come into general use in the behavioral analysis of drug action. Why has the use of these particular techniques become so prevalent?

CONSTANCY OF PROCEDURES

We can begin to answer this question by considering a simple chemical experiment. Suppose we were interested in the relationship of the pressure and the temperature of a gas in a closed vessel. We would, therefore, vary temperature by heating the gas, and then we would measure the resultant pressure. Although we would obtain an orderly relationship between the two variables, comparable results would not be obtained in another laboratory unless the volume of the vessel were the same as the one we had used.

This example seems ridiculously obvious because we know that both temperature and volume interact to determine pressure. The point is nonetheless a vital one: Phenomena cannot be analyzed in the absence of procedures that are constant from experiment to experiment and from laboratory to laboratory. In this case, the orderly relationship called Boyle's law would not have emerged if, first, volume had not been recognized as a significant variable, and second, it had not been held constant from experiment to experiment.

The determinants of behavior are vastly more complex than those involved in Boyle's law. As we shall see again and again, a myriad of factors can determine the behavioral effect of a drug. Thus, we cannot hope to analyze these effects without first identifying relevant variables and then holding them constant. An example involving the drug amphetamine will amplify the point.

Suppose we are interested in the effect amphetamine may have on motor activity. We could reasonably study this effect by using laboratory rats and placing them in a Y-shaped maze. We could record the numbers of times the animals entered the arms of the Y as they moved about the maze; an increased number of entries into the arms could sensibly be supposed to reflect an increase in motor activity. Amphetamine has been studied in this way, and Robbins (1977) has provided us with a survey of the available data. Six studies were surveyed; all used the Y-maze procedure we have just considered. The procedures seem comparable, simple, and straightforward, yet only two studies reported increased activity due to amphetamine, whereas two reported no effect of drug, and two others, a decrease in activity.

In one sense, this array of all possible outcomes is not surprising because, as we shall see, differences in procedure can determine drug effect. On the other hand, the variety of results is unexpected because the Y-maze procedures seem to be essentially the same. But they are not; relevant factors must have been different in the different studies.

What might some of the salient factors that generally determine behavioral outcome actually be? Can the relevant variables be identified so that they can be held constant? A partial listing of such factors is given in Table 2–2.

Of the ten factors listed, our concern here is with the tenth. Thus, we want to be able to hold the other factors constant, just as we held volume constant in studying the relationship of temperature (analogous to drug) and pressure (analogous to behavioral effect). And that is what the procedures we have discussed do provide: Level of noise and illumination are constant; extraneous noise is minimized by the use of a sound-attenuating chamber for the animal; chamber size is roughly constant; the response required (e.g., lever depression) is the same in all experiments; strain, sex, and species of animal are not varied; schedules of reinforcement are rigidly defined; and type of reinforcement can be held constant. Furthermore, these procedures employ automatic equipment for the control of stimuli and reinforcements presented to the animal. Accordingly, there is a procedural constancy that cannot be obtained with manual control by a human experimenter; people are not as invariant as machines. It is not surprising, therefore, that behavior controlled by an FI schedule, for example, is essentially the same in different experiments. It is also not surprising that reproducible drug effects are also a consequence of this constancy of procedure.

RELIABILITY

In considering the relation of pressure to temperature, we tacitly assumed that our pressure gauge and our thermometer were accurate. But suppose this were not so. If either the pressure gauge or the thermometer did not give the same readings under constant conditions, formulation of a general law about the behavior of gases would not be possible. That is, measuring devices must be reliable.

The term *reliability*, as it is used in this context, refers to agreement

Table 2–2

1. Noise level	6. Species of animal
2. Level of illumination	7. Strain and sex of animal
3. Extraneous sound	8. Schedule of reinforcement
4. Chamber size	9. Type of reinforcement
5. Response required	10. Drug

between measurements. A measurement at one time should be the same as a later reading if experimental conditions have not changed. Without a reliable means of measurement, however, a different reading could mean either that the conditions of the experiment have changed or that the measuring instrument itself has changed.

Lack of agreement between measurements (unreliability) can be due to either the measuring device or to the observer who reads the device and records the reading obtained. There can be instrument errors and there can be observer errors. It is obvious that reproducible results cannot be obtained if both of these sources of error are not minimized.

With respect to the techniques just discussed, such errors have been minimized by the way in which the animal's response is defined and recorded. A response is defined as the closure of a switch; automatic equipment is used to tally these switch closures. There is thus no ambiguity about whether responses occur or about the rate at which they are emitted. (Equipment failure can, of course, occur but is extraordinarily rare and easily detected.) Furthermore, the procedural constancy that we have already considered increases the likelihood that one experimenter will record the same events as another experimenter. This is another reason why the use of these techniques has become so pervasive—they are extremely reliable.

The topic of reliability is also important because it bears on issues other than the use of particular technological procedures; it leads us directly to a consideration of observational procedures.

DIRECT OBSERVATIONS OF BEHAVIOR

We will have occasion to consider some of the problems inherent in observational procedures in discussions of the clinical effects of drugs in later chapters; for the moment we will focus on their use in laboratory contexts.

When we consider direct observations of the behavioral effects of drugs, we are asking an implicit question: Why can we not simply look at an animal's response to drug and report what we observe? There is no inherent reason why we cannot, in fact, do just that. The problem is, rather, that such a procedure makes our studies especially vulnerable to the problems just discussed, for two basic reasons: Direct observations often show poor agreement within an experiment, and they are especially subject to experimental bias.

RELIABILITY

With the method of direct observation, the observer is both the measuring instrument and the recorder of the resultant measurements. The observer becomes, in effect, both the pressure gauge and the one who reads the gauge. Thus, two potential sources of error are combined. We can ask, then, how well do observers agree in their measurements, and how much error is introduced?

As it turns out, empirical studies of observational methods indicate that agreement is rather hard to come by. And it is easy to see why this should be so; the movements of animals often occur quite rapidly, and the view that an observer has of the animal can determine what is actually seen. Furthermore, there may be substantial ambiguity in defining just what constitutes a given response category.

Given those problems, we can ask how well the observers actually do. In studies summarized by Norton (1977), for example, videotapes of animal movements were shown to trained observers to determine the extent to which they agreed on categorizing behavior. The average reliability coefficient was 0.832. What does a coefficient of 0.832 mean about the extent of agreement under these presumably optimal conditions?

In order to answer this question we must imagine that there is a "true" score that can be only approximated by our measurement. Suppose for the moment that, under constant conditions, the "true" pressure in a system is some value called T. Because neither the gauge nor the process of reading it is totally free of error (E), T can never actually be known exactly. What is known is what is observed; observation (O) can be thought of as the sum of the "true" pressure and whatever error there is in the recording system; i.e., $O = T + E$.

Now consider the situation in which observers rate the extent of movement they see on a videotape. The observers can, for example, be asked to assign a number such as 1 to a small movement, a larger value of 2 to a larger movement, a 3 to a still more extensive movement, and so on. Imagine that there are five instances of movement and that the observers are asked to rate these movements to provide estimates (Os) of the T values for each movement. Further suppose that there are two observers, both of whom rate each of the five movements; these ratings supply the data shown in Table 2–3. (Recall that the "true" values are entirely hypothetical and can be only approximated by the observations.)

Table 2–3

True movement	First observer	Second observer
1	2 (1)*	1 (0)
2	2 (0)	3 (1)
3	4 (1)	3 (0)
4	5 (1)	6 (2)
5	6 (1)	5 (0)

* Values of E are given in parentheses.

Each observer provides a score that is equal to $T + E$. If the values of E were zero in all case, then each observer would provide a rating equal to T (i.e., 1, 2, 3, 4, and 5 for both observers). Accordingly, the ratings for the two would agree perfectly. But because there are errors, which are different for each observer, the raters do not agree. In other words, the greater the error, the *less* the agreement.

The reliability coefficient is a way of describing the extent of agreement and thereby of estimating the extent of error. In particular, these coefficients can range from +1.0 through zero to −1.0. A coefficient of +1.0 indicates perfect agreement (no error), whereas a value of zero indicates no agreement (maximum error). (A value of −1.0 indicates perfect *dis*agreement; if one observer assigned a value of 1, the other would assign a 5, a 2 would be paired with 4, and so on. For our purposes, we need consider only positive values of the reliability coefficient.) Looked at in this way, the coefficient of 0.832 that we considered before indicates that there is some error (the coefficient is less than 1.0) but that the error is not maximal (the coefficient is greater than zero). We can, however, get a more precise idea about the meaning of the coefficient by borrowing a concept from engineering. This concept is the **signal-to-noise ratio.**

When we listen to a radio, for example, we hear a signal (the music we want to hear) as well as a certain amount of static (the "noise" we do not want to hear). These outputs are both variations in sound level; their relationship can be expressed as a signal-to-noise ratio (S/N). Obviously, we want this ratio to be high, because if it is not, we have difficulty detecting the signal—hearing the music over the noise.

Both the music and static are variations in output from the radio. Similarly, the T values and O values in Table 2–3 are characterized by variation. We can regard the T values as "signal" (the variation that we want to dectect—analogous to the music) and the errors as "noise." Although we can never actually measure the T values, it can be shown that a signal-to-noise ratio can be obtained for these variations just as they can for the variations in sound. In particular, for a reliability coefficient R, it can be shown that $S/N = R/1 - R$ (see Cronbach, 1970). Thus, if $R = O$, errors ("noise") are maximal and $S/N = O$; we cannot detect the signal (T values) because of the static. On the other hand, as R approaches 1.00, S/N becomes indefinitely large; we have no difficulty in detecting the signal. In our example, $R = 0.832$ and $S/N = 4.952$.

We can get a better sense of the meaning of a S/N ratio of about 5.0 from the following everyday examples: A good hi-fi amplifier has a S/N ratio of about 100. The S/N ratio of a good television is about 100; the picture will be distinctly "snowy" at 30 and quite poor at 10.

When we consider the techniques discussed earlier in this chapter, we realize that the S/N ratios are necessarily very large: There can be virtually no disagreement about the numbers of lever presses that occur in 10 minutes, for example, because these are automatically recorded—because there is very little margin of error. In contrast, coefficients in the range of 0.8 to 0.9 are evidently the maxima for direct observation under optimal circumstances (S/N ratios thus range from 4.0 to 9.0).

We are, of course, interested in detecting behavioral change due to drugs, not in S/N ratios as such. But behavioral change (variation) is the "signal" we want to detect, and the concept of a S/N ratio is thus a useful one because it highlights a major limitation of direct observation: Low S/N ratios mean that our chances of detecting variations due to drug are substantially reduced.

BIAS

An observer can be biased in judgment of behavior; it is well documented that the observer's expectation about what a treatment "should" do can influence the outcome of observation.

There are two general ways in which such bias can be minimized. One of these is by using an observer who knows neither what the drug is nor whether a drug has been given at all. Such an observer is conventionally said to be "blind."

The problem with "blind" observation is that there are two ways in which the observer can "see." In the first place, any trained observer can detect the fact that some drug has been given because "something" is different about the animal's behavior. Furthermore, no drug is devoid of side-effects, and many of these are easily observed. Thus, an observer who has a knowledge of drug action—and most do—is likely to be able to make a nonrandom guess of what the drug actually is. At the very least, there can be an expectation that shifts the observation away from what would be obtained from a truly unbiased observer. (Drugs that produce salivation, for example, are more likely to have certain behavioral effects than those that do not.) Thus, it is extraordinarily difficult to find an observer who is truly "blind." If the biases introduced in different laboratories vary, reproducibility will be reduced.

A second way of minimizing bias involves reducing the role of expectation in producing bias: It is unlikely that different observers will have precisely the same expectations. Therefore, as the number of observers is increased, the role of systematic bias will tend to be reduced. In Table 2–3, for example, both observers are biased in that both tend to overestimate the T values; this communality of bias reflects the realistic likelihood that there will be some shared expectation. However, the first observer is more biased (average error = 4/5 = 0.8) than the second (average error = 3/5 = 0.6). Combining observations from the two would therefore introduce less bias (average error = 7/10 = 0.7) than that involved if only the first observer's ratings were used.

These considerations lead us to expect two things: that more than one observer would be routinely used in behavioral studies involving direct observation and that a measure of their agreement would be reported. Surprisingly results of a survey by Poling, Cleary, and Monaghan (1980) indicate that this is definitely not the case: Of the 4000 articles surveyed, fewer than 5% provided a measure of interobserver agreement; equally surprising is the finding that fewer than 10% of the studies surveyed used a "blind" observer. These shortcomings are not, of course, intrinsic to observational methods themselves but to the ways in which they are evidently used.

The problems of bias and reliability should not, in any case, be taken to indicate that observational procedures are useless. Indeed, these procedures can provide important insights into the character of pharmacologic effect and, looked at in this way, can be said to have been underutilized. The fact remains, however, that they can be especially vulnerable to the problems of reliability and potential bias, whereas the other procedures discussed provide for great interexperiment consistancy, extremely high reliability, and an absence of bias in the measurement process. These facts undoubtedly account for their prevalent use in the behavioral analysis of drug action. And because these procedures have become dominant, it is with them that the vast majority of experimental data in behavioral pharmacology have been accumulated. We must, therefore, turn to them as we examine behavioral pharmacology in the chapters that lie ahead.

NOTES

1. Discriminated avoidance is sometimes referred to as "classical avoidance," presumably because it has a procedural similarity to the "classical conditioning" procedures developed by Pavlov. In the Pavlovian technique, however, shock is delivered regardless of whether or not the animal has responded during the preceding signal.

   The fact that an avoidance contingency is absent in the Pavlovian technique introduces an important difference that is blurred by the use of one word to refer to two very different procedures. The usage is ill-advised.

2. When an animal has moved from the left-hand compartment to the right-hand one, it is necessarily required to return to the left-hand compartment on the next trial. If the animal was shocked in the left-hand compartment, then, on the succeeding trial, it is faced with the prospect of returning to the very place in which shock was previously delivered.

   This feature of two-way avoidance thus incorporates an aspect of the punishment procedures that will be discussed shortly. And, as we shall see, punishment tends to suppress ongoing behavior; such suppression interferes, in turn, with the active response required of the animal if it is to avoid. Looked at in this way, two-way avoidance is a very complicated affair, not a simple variant on the one-way procedure.

3. Another feature of both one-way and two-way discriminated avoidance is that the animal may emit "unauthorized" responses in the intervals between presentation of the warning signals. This fact provides another behavioral index that may be affected by drug independently of, or in addition to, any effect the drug may have on avoidance and escape responding themselves.

4. There is one other procedure that should be briefly noted. It involves *non*reinforcement and is labeled **extinction** (EXT). If an animal has previously been trained to respond on some schedule of reinforce-

ment, for example, the device for delivering reinforcements can then be disconnected so that responding is never reinforced. The introduction of EXT would, of course, eventually produce a cessation of responding. But animals do not abruptly stop responding immediately following the introduction of EXT; instead, they may continue to respond for substantial periods of time in a way that is determined by their prior history of reinforcement (see Ferster and Skinner, 1957).

Chapter 3

Basic
Pharmacologic
Procedures

IN THIS CHAPTER we will consider a variety of pharmacologic techniques relevant to the analysis of drug action. We will be concerned with two general topics: first, the ways in which drugs can be administered, and second, the kinds of information that are necessary for an adequate analysis of drug action.

ROUTES OF DRUG ADMINISTRATION

The most common way in which drugs are administered is by mouth, designated as **p.o.** (from the Latin *per os*). But drugs can be, and have been, given by all conceivable routes, ranging from nasal to rectal. In most experimental procedures, however, three routes in addition to p.o. are the most commonly used: One of these is intravenous, directly into the vein; it is noted as **i.v.** Another widely used route involves injection into the peritoneal cavity, that space below the diaphram that houses stomach, intestines, and all the rest; this is the intraperitoneal route, designated as **i.p.** The last route commonly used is the intramuscular route, noted as **i.m.**—the route for most of the "shots" given for inoculation.

These different routes can produce differences in drug effect because of differences in absorption and passage into the bloodstream (e.g., onset of activity is much more rapid following i.v. than i.p. or p.o. administration). As a general rule, however, these differences are minor ones.

THE DOSE–RESPONSE FUNCTION

The word "function" as used in analysis refers to a relationship between two variables. This relationship is usually described by some equation that in turn can be portrayed in graphic form. For example, body weight is a function of food intake; the particulars of the relationship can be represented as a curve.

Analysis of drug action invariably includes determination of the dose–response function. The two variables that define this function are dose of drug and corresponding behavioral effect. The dose—or amount—is usually expressed in milligrams (mg) relative to the body weight of the recipient in kilograms (kg). That is, dose is usually expressed in **mg/kg** units.[1]

Behavioral effect is expressed in a wide variety of ways, as we shall see as we proceed. Despite this variation, all indices of behavioral effect are designed to reflect a single concern: whether behavior is increased or decreased by drug. The dose–response function is, then, an expression of the nature of the behavioral change induced by differing doses of drug.

THE BIPHASIC DOSE–RESPONSE FUNCTION

Virtually all of the drugs that we shall be considering have biphasic effects. That is, low doses produce behavioral increments, whereas relatively higher ones produce decrements.

The curve for one such function is shown at the top of Figure 3–1. It shows that, as dose is increased, the behavioral effect being measured first increases gradually, then levels off, and finally declines. The initial level of responding, the control level that occurs without drug, is indicated by the horizontal dashed line.

Suppose that for study of a certain drug, we happen to choose the amount (dose) at *A* in the figure; our conclusion would be that the drug is biologically **inactive** or inert—does nothing—because the level of responding following drug administration is not different from the control level. But suppose we happened to choose the dose at *B*; we would conclude that the drug is a **stimulant**—it increases behavioral output relative to initial level. With the dose at *C,* we would conclude that the drug is a **depressant**—it reduces level of responding.

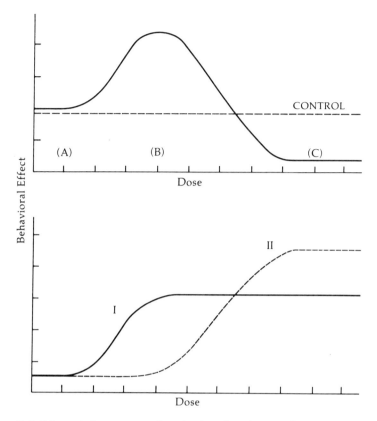

Figure 3–1. Schematic dose–response function for a drug that initially increases responding (top). The hypothetical effect of different doses on two incompatible behaviors is shown at the bottom. (The levels of *I* and *II* would ultimately decline at higher doses; i.e., both would be characterized by a dose–response function like that shown at the top of the figure.)

All three statements are true; yet none characterizes the drug. The drug is, in fact, all three—inactive, a stimulant, and a depressant. This is not merely a hypothetical possibility: *Any* drug that initially produces an incremental effect can show the kind of pattern depicted at the top of Figure 3–1, although the relative rates of rise and decline in effect may differ. Thus, it is obviously impossible to characterize a drug on the basis of a single dose.

Interpretation of Depressant Effects When a drug produces a decrease in responding (as at *C*), it is often assumed that such an effect represents a generalized decrement in all categories of behavior. This may be the case: The animal may be motorically incapacitated, asleep, or, as a limiting case, dead. On the other hand, a decrement may reflect not a general "depression" but an increase in some behavior that is incompatible with the behavior being measured. This possibility is schematized at the bottom of Figure 3–1.

Measurement of a certain behavior (*I* in the figure) might show that increases in dose of drug increased that behavior to a maximum beyond which there was no further increment in the dose range under study. Measurement of a second behavior (*II*) might demonstrate the same relationship except that higher doses of drug were required. But now suppose that the behaviors were incompatible—that *II* interfered with *I*. The net result of an increase in behavior *II* would be a decline in behavior *I* (as shown at the top of Figure 3–1 for doses greater than *B*). The following example illustrates the point:

Relatively low doses of the drug amphetamine given to a rat increase generalized locomotion; higher doses produce an increase in sniffing and gnawing. In the rat, these latter behaviors occur while the animal is in one place. Thus, an increase in their occurrence (due to high doses of drug) interferes with locomotion in space.

If, following amphetamine administration, all movement regardless of type (locomotion, sniffing, gnawing, and so forth), were rerecorded, movement would be found to increase with increasing dose of drug. If only locomotion were measured, however, increasing doses would produce an increase followed by a decline (as at the top of Figure 3–1). But the decline does not reflect a generalized decrement; rather, it is due to an increase in another behavior. In other words, "less" can be a consequence of "more." Thus, what we observe will be a consequence of what we happen to measure.

This point is one we shall encounter again and again: The behavioral effect of a drug cannot be divorced from the way in which that effect is measured. In the case diagrammed at the top of Figure 3–1, the depressant effect (at dose *C*) could reflect either a generalized decrement or a stimulant action that has not been measured. Thus, labeling a drug a "stimulant" or a "depressant" is at best a very crude classification. More to the point, such labeling in the absence of a specification of the behavior being measured can be very misleading, as we shall see.

Different Doses—Two Drugs   Now consider a comparison of two drugs. The dose–response functions for the two (*I* and *II*) are shown in Figure 3–2. If we chose dose *A*, we would conclude that drug *I* is more of a stimulant than drug *II*—which is true at those equal doses. But if we chose dose *B*, we would conclude just the opposite; drug *II* is more of a stimulant than drug *I*. If we chose dose *C*, however, we would decide that both drugs are depressants and that drug *I* is more depressant than drug *II*. All of these conclusions are correct for the individual doses. Collectively, they make no sense:

1. At dose *A*, *I* is a stimulant and *II* is not.
2. At dose *B*, *II* is a stimulant and *I* is not (contradicts 1, above).
3. At dose *C*, both *I* and *II* are depressants (contradicts both 1 and 2, above).

Drug *I* can be said to be relatively more **potent** than drug *II* in that increases in behavior are obtained at lower doses, as are decrements. Thus, there is a quantitative but not a qualitative difference between the two.

In considering Figure 3–2, we were concerned with only two drugs and a single measured behavior. But now suppose that two *behaviors*, not drugs, were measured.

Different Doses of One Drug—Two Behaviors   No drug has a single effect on behavior or, for that matter, on any biologic process. This point can be illustrated by considering only two behavioral indices and the effect of one drug. Refer to Figure 3–2 again, but in this instance, let *I* and *II* represent two behaviors, not drugs.

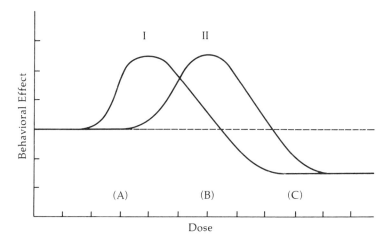

Figure 3–2. Schematic dose–response functions for the effects of two different drugs (*I* and *II*) on one behavior. The figure can also be used to describe the effects of one drug on two different behaviors (see text).

If the dose of the single drug were *A,* we would conclude that this drug increased behavior *I* but had no effect on behavior *II*—in effect, that the action of the drug was specific to behavior *I.* With dose *B*, on the other hand, we would have concluded exactly the opposite. But had the tests of behavioral effect been carried out over a range of doses (from zero to *B*, say) we would correctly conclude that the drug can increase behavior and that behavior *I* is relatively more sensitive than behavior *II.*

It is true that the drug can increase behavior, and that different behaviors have differential sensitivities to this effect. It is also true that the drug can *decrease* the very same behaviors, a fact that emerges only if a complete range of doses is evaluated.

Behavioral Determinants and Drug Effect   The following experiment, of considerable historical importance, provides a good example of variability in pharmacologic effect not attributable to drug or dose. Dews (1955) trained pigeons to respond to either an FR or an FI schedule. Once performance had stabilized on either of the schedules, the birds were given the drug pentobarbital in varying doses (expressed as mg/kg and given i.m.).

Pentobarbital will be discussed more fully later; for the moment we need consider only Dews' general findings, summarized in Figure 3–3. The horizontal dashed line indicates the control levels of responding obtained after control (saline) injections; the plotted values are differences from these control levels for FI responding (the solid line) and for FR responding (the dashed line).

The effect of drug depends on the measure of behavior. Consider the effect of 1.0 mg/kg: pentobarbital is both a depressant (as far as FI behavior is concerned) and a stimulant (as far as FR behavior is concerned). Pentobarbital and drugs like it are traditionally classed as depressants, but are they? The answer depends on both the dose and the behavior studied. Pentobarbital is a depressant at 1.0 mg/kg if behavior maintained by FI is the measure; it is a stimulant at this same dose if FR responding is the measure. At higher doses it produces a greater depressant effect on FI than on FR responding (compare Figure 3–2).

Comparable phenomena are evident in data that we considered in the preceding chapter (Figure 2–10). In that instance, a dose of ethanol (e.g., 1.5 g/kg) that decreased FI responding (when the opposite component was FR60) also *in*creased FI responding (when the opposite component was FR 150).

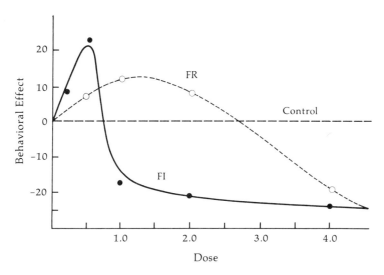

Figure 3–3. Differential effects of pentobarbital on responding maintained by an FI schedule of reinforcement as compared to that maintained by an FR schedule. (Redrawn from Dews, 1955).

Data like these make a very important general point: the variables controlling behavior enter into the determination of pharmacologic effect just as the kind of drug and its dose do. It is impossible to characterize pharmacologic activity without also specifying the interaction of drug, dose, *and* the determinants of the behavior being measured. This rule about interactions is not a reflection of some laboratory curiosity—as a matter of fact, such interactions occur in everyday experience. Both alcohol and marijuana, for example, are both characterized as depressants, yet both are described as producing a "high." Such effects can vary profoundly as a function of context—two martinis are very likely to have different effects in different circumstances (e.g., solitary drinking versus a cocktail party). Thus, the basic ideas generated by the procedures we have been considering are not essentially different from what can be observed in ordinary experience. What *is* different about these procedures is that the variables controlling differential effects can be specified, systematically varied, and thereby analyzed in a way that is not possible with procedures that depend on casual observation.

THE MONOPHASIC DOSE–RESPONSE FUNCTION

As already noted, virtually all of the drugs that we shall be considering have biphasic effects; behavior is increased at low doses and necessarily decreased at high ones. A few drugs, however, have only decremental effects. But this fact does not modify the crucial importance of determining dose–response functions in analyzing behavioral effect, for two reasons.

In the first place, whether a dose–response function is monophasic or biphasic cannot be known unless the effects of a wide range of doses are examined—unless the dose–response function is first determined. Clearly, studying only a single dose would not reveal whether the decremental effects obtained were characteristic of all doses or were a reflection of the action of a high dose in an otherwise biphasic function (e.g., dose C in Figure 3–1).

Similarly, comparison of single doses of two drugs could erroneously suggest that one drug is inactive simply because the dose chosen was too low. That is, both drugs could actually be characterized by decrementing monophasic functions, but this could not be determined in the absence of complete dose–response determinations for both.

Thus, the adequate characterization of a single drug or the comparison of two drugs always involves dose–response determination.

THE THERAPEUTIC RATIO AND ITS EXTENSION

The dose-dependency characteristic of drug effects leads directly to the concept of the *therapeutic ratio*. This ratio incorporates the idea of differential dose-dependencies into a single number. The value of this number, used in pharmacologic analysis to indicate the safety of a drug, is the quotient of two numerical indices of drug effect called the ED_{50} and the LD_{50}—that is, ED_{50}/LD_{50}.

The ED_{50}—median effective dose—is the dose (D) of drug that is effective (E) in 50% of the animals tested. (This value can be estimated in several ways that depend on the particulars of the experiment. For our purposes, we need note only that it indicates a dose of "average" effectiveness for a particular effect of a particular drug. Thus, if the ED_{50} of one drug in producing a given effect is lower than a second drug in producing the same effect, the former is said to be more potent in producing that effect.) The LD_{50}—median lethal dose—is a comparable index that refers to the dose (D) that is lethal (L) for 50% of the animals. Thus, the ratio of these two indicates how safe a drug is because, as the ED_{50} value approaches the LD_{50} value (i.e., ED_{50}/LD_{50} approaches 1.0), the effect in question cannot be obtained without running the risk of death. Conversely, as the therapeutic ratio decreases (ED_{50}/LD_{50} less than 1.0), safety *increases* because the effect can be obtained at doses lower than the average lethal dose.

The therapeutic ratio reflects the relative potencies of a drug with respect to an issue of obvious clinical significance: the production of a given effect relative to toxicity. For example, a drug that induces sleep but has a high therapeutic ratio will be less safe and, therefore, generally less useful than one with a low ratio.

The logic of the therapeutic ratio can be extended to comparisons involving other spectra of activity. For example, suppose in the analysis of a certain drug we obtain a dose-dependent continuum that shows it to increase responding at low doses and to decrease it at higher doses (e.g., the effects of pentobarbital in Figure 3–3). We can estimate the ED_{50} for both of these effects—that is, the ED_{50}-I and ED_{50}-D for response increment and decrement, respectively. Suppose we have a second drug that has the same biphasic action; we can estimate the ED_{50}-I and ED_{50}-D for this drug also. We can now compare these two drugs in three ways.

First, the magnitudes of the two ED_{50}-I values will tell us that the drug with the lower value is the more potent in producing increases in responding. Second, the ED_{50}-D values will tell us which is the more potent in producing response decrement. Note that the drug that is more potent in increasing responding (the drug with the lower ED_{50}-I) need not be the more potent in decreasing responding; this will depend on the form of the dose–response functions for the two drugs.

Finally, the ratios of the ED_{50}-I to the ED_{50}-D values for each of the drugs will tell us which drug increases responding over the wider range. Generally speaking, the lower the ratio of ED_{50}-I to ED_{50}-D, the wider the range of the response-increasing capacity of the drug. These ratios are themselves *relative* measures; the ratios themselves, *relative* to each other, can differentiate the drugs. It is not enough to say that one is a stimulant or a depressant, because both drugs could be either. The differentiation is an entirely relative affair.[2]

A HYPOTHETICAL EXAMPLE: BIPHASIC FUNCTION

For further clarification of ED_{50}s and ratios, consider the values in Table 3–1 for two hypothetical drugs, Drug I and Drug II. The values at (a) are the control response levels obtained when a control injection of saline is given. A dose of Drug I at 1.0 mg/kg (b) reliably increases responding, whereas a dose of 4.0 mg/kg (c) reliably decreases it. Such a dose is called the **minimum effective dose,** abbreviated **MED**; the lowest dose that reliably increases behavior is called **MED-I,** and the lowest dose that reliably decreases it, **MED-D.**

The values for Drug II present a slightly more complicated picture. The lowest dose that reliably increases responding (MED-I) is somewhere between the control value of 100 and the value obtained at 1.0 mg/kg (d). By interpolation, the dose required to produce a response level of 110 would be halfway between the control level and this latter value. Thus, as shown in Table 3–2, the estimated MED-I for Drug II is 0.5 mg/kg (b); the MED-D for this same drug is 8.0 mg/kg (d).

The data in Table 3–2 tell us that Drug II is *more* potent than Drug I in increasing responding. That is, the MED-I is lower for Drug II than for Drug I; compare (a) and (b). However, Drug II is *less* potent in decreasing responding; compare (c) and (d).

The fact that the ratio for Drug II is less than that for Drug I—compare (e) and (f)—tells us that response increments can be obtained over a wider dose range with Drug II than with Drug I. (Analogously, if the values for the MED-Ds were actually LD values, Drug II would have the lower therapeutic ratio and would therefore be the safer drug.)

These numbers can be confusing because low values do not indicate less potency or effectiveness, as might be expected. Remember an "upside-down" rule: The *lower* the MED (or ED), the *greater* the potency; the *lower* the relative ratio, the *greater* the range of effectiveness.

Table 3–1

Dose (mg/kg)	Percentage Control	
	Drug I	Drug II
0 (a)	100	100
1	110 (b)	120 (d)
2	150	250
4	90 (c)	120
8	60	90 (e)

Table 3–2

Value	Drug I	Drug II
MED-I	1.000 (a)	0.500 (b)
MED-D	4.000 (c)	8.000 (d)
MED-I/MED-D	0.250 (e)	0.062 (f)

AN EXAMPLE OF A MONOPHASIC FUNCTION: THE NEUROLEPTICS

Later, we will consider the effects of a class of drugs that is used in the management of psychotic behavior in humans (the so-called neuroleptic drugs). These drugs have the property of reducing discriminated avoidance responding of the kind discussed in Chapter 2; they can also reduce escape responding—the responding that can occur when there has been a failure to avoid shock.

Any other drug can decrease these two classes of behavior. Yet the effects of the neuroleptics on avoidance and escape distinguish this group from the others. They do so not because of qualitative differences among the drugs but because of relative differences among them. In particular, the dose of neuroleptic required to decrease avoidance responding is much smaller than that required to decrease escape behavior; the relative measure of these two effects (the ratio of the doses) is thus small. The comparable relative measures for the other drugs is large and, in most cases, approaches 1.0 (e.g., avoidance and escape are comparably reduced at nearly the same doses).

The hypothetical data in Figure 3–4 illustrate the point. The curves shown in Figure 3–4A depict dose–response functions for two behaviors (*I* and *II*). If these behaviors were avoidance (*I*) and escape (*II*) in a discriminated avoidance situation, the separation of the functions would be typical of the neuroleptics. That is, percent avoidance falls much more rapidly with increasing dose than does percent escape.[3]

A common and useful way of describing dose–response functions is to plot behavioral change in relation to the logarithm of drug dose. The curves shown in Figure 3–4B are plotted in this way; the actual values are the same as those shown in Figure 3–4A.

One advantage of a logarithmic plot is that it amplifies the effects obtained at low doses. Thus, the ED_{50} for avoidance is clearly 10.0 mg/kg, as indicated by the arrows that intersect the solid line. Similarly, the ED_{50} for escape can be obtained by extending the arrow from 50% to the dashed line and extrapolating to the baseline (the ED_{50} is 100.0 mg/kg). The ratio of these two ED_{50} values is analogous to a therapeutic ratio and, in this case, equals 0.100 (10/100).

The hypothetical dose–response data plotted in Figure 3–4C are for a second drug. The values for *avoidance* responding are the same as those in Figure 3–4A and 4B; the ED_{50} is thus 10.0 mg/kg in this case as well. The ED_{50} for *escape* is 16.0 mg/kg. The ratio of ED_{50} values is therefore 0.625 (10/16).

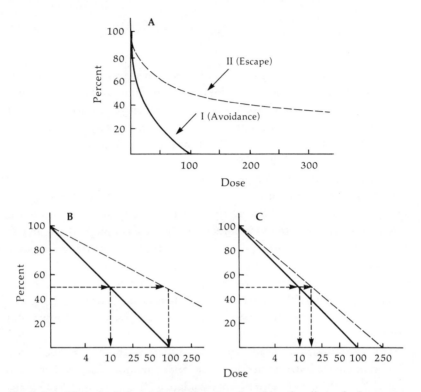

Figure 3–4. Monophasic dose–response functions describing the effects of a drug on two classes of responding in a discriminated avoidance procedure (escape and avoidance). The doses shown in *A* are plotted on a linear coordinate, whereas those in *B* and *C* are plotted logarithmically. The effects in *C* differ from those in *A* and *B* only in that decrements in escape responding occur at lower doses.

On the basis of these ratios, the drug shown in Figure 3–4A and B has a more selective effect than does the drug shown in Figure 3–4C. That is, in the first case, avoidance behavior is decreased at a much lower dose than that necessary for decreasing escape responding (low ratio); this separation is much less in the second case (higher ratio). In fact, according to the relative dose-dependent effects of these two drugs, the selectivity of the first is greater than that of the second by a factor of more than 6 (0.625/0.100 = 6.250).

Now consider the values plotted in Figure 3–5A. There is not much to distinguish these data from those shown in Figure 3–4A. However, when the same values are replotted on logarithmic dose coordinates (Figure 3–5B), a very different picture emerges (compare Figure 3–4B). In this case, the ED_{50} values are the same (10.0 mg/kg for avoidance and 100.0 mg/kg for escape), but the relationship of the dose–response functions is obviously very different.

Three points can be made about Figure 3–5: First, it illustrates the utility of the logarithmic plot in clarifying dose–response functions. Second, it makes it clear that descriptive values like the ED_{50} or MED—useful as they are—cannot fully characterize important differences in these functions; the ED_{50} values for I and II in Figure 3–5B are

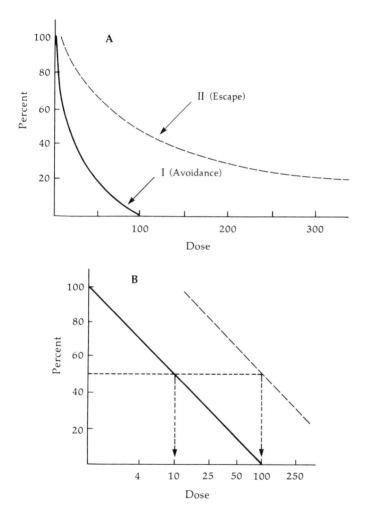

Figure 3–5. Monophasic dose–response functions describing the effects of a drug on two classes of responding. The doses in A are plotted on a linear coordinate, whereas those in B are plotted logarithmically. (Compare Figure 3–4A with Figure 3–5A and Figure 3–4B with Figure 3–5B.)

identical to those in Figure 3–4B, yet the functions obviously differ from each other.

Third and last, the functions in Figure 3–4B have different slopes, indicating that behavior I is more **sensitive** to increasing dose than is behavior *II*. Another way of looking at this differential sensitivity is in terms of the degree of behavioral change due to a constant increase in dose: behavior *I* changes more than behavior *II* as a consequence of the same increase in dosage. (In the increment from 10.0 mg/kg to 100.00 mg/kg, for example, behavior *I* shifts from 50% to zero, whereas behavior *II* shifts from 75% to 50%.)

In contrast, the two behaviors characterized in Figure 3–5B do not differ in overall sensitivity; the dose–response functions do not differ in slope—they are parallel. Rather, the difference in ED_{50} values hinges on the fact that behavior *II* is totally *in*sensitive to doses less than 10.0 mg/kg. This relationship indicates that there is a difference in the **threshold** dose characteristic of the two behaviors; the threshold for behavior II is at 10.0 mg/kg, so that doses less than this are without effect.

These differences bear on the way in which the differential effects of different drugs on different behaviors are conceptualized, and at a more general level, they again illustrate a crucial point: Just as dose–response specification is necessary for the characterization of the effects of different drugs on a single behavior, it is also necessary for the characterization of the effect of a single drug on different behaviors.

DRUG–RECEPTOR INTERACTIONS

The two most striking features of drug action are potency and specificity. Following ingestion of an aspirin tablet, for example, very few milligrams of drug actually reach the brain, yet this is enough to reduce headache. That is, drugs are very potent; a little goes a long way.

Drugs are also specific in their actions. Insulin lowers blood sugar levels, for example, but aspirin does not; aspirin can reduce headache, but insulin does not. These facts suggest that drugs do not act on cells in a random, hit-or-miss fashion; rather, certain drugs act on certain cells. Drug action is highly selective.

CHEMICAL CONFORMATION IN SPECIFICITY AND POTENCY

The selectivity involved in drug action suggests that different cells have receptors for which certain drugs have a high affinity. One way of conceptualizing such affinity is to recognize that each drug has a specific chemical structure with a particular spatial conformation. It is thus reasonable to suppose that different receptors have different conformations that complement the conformations characteristic of different drugs. Receptors are, by analogy, different "locks" into which a very few "keys" (drugs) fit. When a particular "key" does fit a particular "lock," pharmacologic activity results.

Figure 3–6 provides a schematic representation of some drug–receptor interactions. Structures of four different drugs (A through D), each with a different conformation, are schematized at the top of the figure. Each of these has the potential to interact with a certain receptor, as indicated by the arrows. The consequence of each of these interactions is shown at the bottom of the figure.[4]

The receptor is depicted as having three sites, two of which produce behavioral activity; these active sites are indicated as *1* and *2*. A drug that can occupy these sites, with resulting pharmacologic activity, is cal-

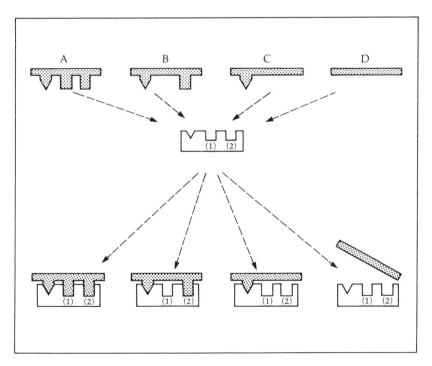

Figure 3–6. Schematic representation of different drug–receptor interactions. Drugs A and B are agonists, drug C is an antagonist, and drug D is inactive (see text for details).

led an **agonist**. Drug A in the figure can occupy both sites and therefore produces maximal activity. Drug B is also an agonist but can occupy only one active site; it thus produces only partial activity and is therefore less potent than drug A.

Drug C can occupy neither of the active sites but does have an affinity for the receptor in the sense that it does "fit" an inactive site. Such a drug is called an **antagonist** because, although it does not itself produce activity, it will block the access of agonists to the receptor. An antagonist is thus roughly analogous to a key that can be inserted into a lock, does not turn the bolt, but does block a key that would work.

Drug D has a conformation that characterizes the vast majority of drugs in relation to a particular receptor. It is neither an agonist nor an antagonist.

A variant on this theme is shown in Figure 3–7. The structure of drug A is again schematized at the top of the figure; in this case the drug can act on either of two receptors, both of which have two active sites. The drug–receptor interaction shown at the left will produce a maximum effect. On the other hand, the same drug has a lowered affinity for the receptor at the right and will produce a reduced effect in interaction with it.

Activities at different receptors, like the two schematized in Figure 3–7, produce different behavioral effects. Thus, as the figure indicates, a single drug can generate different behavioral consequences (Effect I versus Effect II). It is a mistake to think in terms of "one drug–one receptor," because *no* drug has a single behavioral effect; each drug produces a particular **spectrum** of activity. Two such spectra are shown at the bottom of Figure 3–7.

Drug A is maximally active in producing Effect I, as indicated by the arrow on the abscissa. But it does produce activity at other receptors. It will, therefore, produce other effects even though it will be less potent in doing so (as at the receptor on the right, on which only one active site is occupied). Similarly, drug B (from Figure 3–6) has a different spectrum that overlaps with that of A because of a communality of receptor affinity. (Note that drug B is necessarily less potent than drug A with regard to Effect I, as indicated by the arrow on the abscissa.)

Yet another drug (like E) has a spectrum completely divorced from the characteristics of A and B. Thus, drugs do have selective effects (A is not equivalent to E), but this does not mean each drug has only one activity. And, because they do not, different drugs may have overlapping spectra (e.g., A and B) in which their potencies in producing

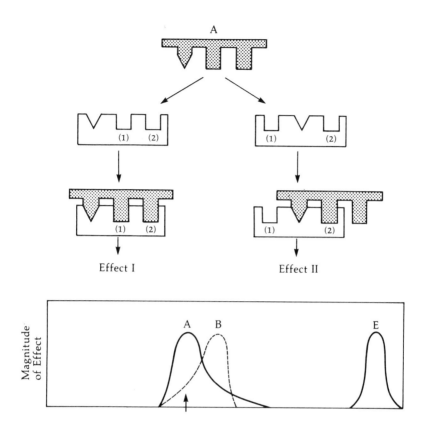

Different Behavioral Effects

Figure 3–7. A schematic representation of the interaction of a drug with two receptors is shown at the top of the figure. The different spectra of behavioral activity produced by different drugs (*A, B,* and *E*) acting at different receptors is shown at the bottom; of the different behavioral effects shown in this schematic, the arrow denotes Effect I.

different effects will differ. This is why, of course, dose–response data are so crucial in differentiating among different drugs.[5]

DRUGS AS MIMICS OF ENDOGENOUS SUBSTANCES: THE EXAMPLE OF ACETYLCHOLINE

Why should there be specific receptors at all? The answer is that receptors have evolved so that cells can be selectively sensitive to the naturally occurring, endogenous chemicals involved in regulating biologic function within the body. Drugs can be said to be "foreign" chemicals that "trick" receptors that have evolved to be selectively sensitive not to alien drugs but to endogenous chemicals. One such endogenous chemical is acetylcholine.

Acetylcholine (ACH) is a naturally occurring substance that is involved in the control of a wide variety of biologic functions, including activity in the brain. There is no doubt that there are ACH receptors, and that some drugs can mimic the actions of ACH at these receptors. Such drugs are agonists that are also called **cholinomimetics** *(cholin* in such combined forms always refers to acetyl*choline)*—they "mime" the effects of ACH. Refer back to Figure 3–6: The conformation labeled *A* corresponds to ACH itself, whereas *B* schematizes the conformation of a cholinomimetic drug.

The conformation labeled *C* in Figure 3–6 is an antagonist at the ACH receptor and, in this context, is called an **anticholinergic**—it produces a blockade of cholinergic (ACH-controlled) function.

ACH ACTIVITY AND ANTICHOLINERGIC EFFECTS

There is a great number of drugs known to have anticholinergic activity. In fact, most of the drugs that we will encounter in Chapters 12 through 17 have some degree of such activity. Let us now consider briefly these anticholinergic effects.[6]

ACH produces two general classes of effect. One of these is called **nicotinic** because similar effects are produced by the well-known drug nicotine. Thus, the ACH receptor that leads to one spectrum of activity can be "tricked" by an alien substance, nicotine. (Nicotine would thus correspond to Drug *B* in Figure 3–6.)

The second class of ACH activity is mimicked by the effects of another drug, muscarine. This spectrum of activity is therefore called **muscarinic.** The ACH receptor that controls this second class of activity can thus be "tricked" by the drug muscarine. ACH therefore acts at two conceptually different receptors, each characterized by a specific conformation; the one defined by nicotine is nicotinic, whereas the second, defined by muscarine, is muscarinic.

Strictly speaking, the term *anticholinergic* could refer to an ACH antagonist that functions at a nicotinic receptor *or* at a muscarinic receptor. However, general usage has evolved so that the term refers only to antagonism of the muscarinic effects of ACH. This usage, not entirely accurate, has apparently become common because the majority of drugs that do have anticholinergic activity antagonize muscarinic effects.[7]

The standard anticholinergics of this type are atropine and scopolamine. They produce, of course, effects opposite to those controlled by

ACH activity at the muscarinic receptor. The effects of both atropine and scopolamine thus include decreased salivation, increased heart rate, dilation of the pupils, reduced sweating, and loss of muscle tone in the bladder and gastrointestinal tract.[8]

Thus, a drug characterized as having anticholinergic effects is an agent that, unless specified otherwise, produces some or all of the effects of atropine or scopolamine. We will encounter a variety of such drugs in later chapters.

NOTES

1. The doses of drugs given to humans are often specified in absolute terms without any specifications of body weight. As a rough rule, the mg/kg level can be obtained by assuming that the average human body weight is 70 kg. (Useful procedures for comparing dose levels for different species have been discussed by Dews and deWeese, 1977).

2. The relative values of ED_{50}-I and ED_{50}-D can be used to compare behavioral measures rather than drugs. For example, if the ED_{50}-I for one measure were lower than that for a second measure, the first measure would be more sensitive to the action of the drug in question. (In Figure 3–3, FI is more sensitive to the incremental effects of pentobarbital than is FR. It is also much more sensitive to the decremental effects of this drug.) Curiously, systematic comparisons of this kind have not been widely used.

3. Data like those shown in Figure 3–4A are sometimes presented as a "percent inhibition." These values thus provide an index of the relative decrement in behavior due to drug and are obtained by calculating the following ratio:

$$\frac{\text{Response level before drug} - \text{Response level after drug}}{\text{Response level before drug}} \times 100$$

The data in Figure 3–4A indicate that the inhibition (or decrement) of avoidance responding is maximal at the 100 mg/kg dose level (100%), whereas the inhibition of escape responding is only 50%.

4. It is important to recognize that this conceptual schematization of drug–receptor interactions vastly oversimplifies the complex biochemical activity that actually takes place in cells.

5. An excellent introductory discussion of the mathematical character-

ization of drug–receptor interactions and how these determine dose–response functions is available in Tallarida and Jacob (1979).

6. Naturally occurring substances are inactivated in the presence of enzymes. Thus, a drug that inhibits these enzymes can increase their activity and thereby produce an indirect agonism. ACH, for example, is inactivated by the enzyme cholinesterase. A drug (e.g., physostigmine) that is a cholinesterase inhibitor will therefore be a cholinergic agonist because it decreases the normal breakdown of ACH and thereby increases and prolongs ACH activity.

7. The usage is an unfortunate one because it seems to imply that the antimuscarinic activity of drugs is somehow more important than their antinicotinic action, which is not at all the case. Strictly speaking, drugs should be characterized as antimuscarinic or antinicotinic, not nonspecifically as anticholinergic. Be that as it may, "anticholinergic" has generally come to mean "antimuscarinic" unless otherwise specified.

8. Two drugs that are closely related to atropine and to scopolamine are methyl atropine and methyl scopolamine. (As their names imply, they differ from the parent compounds by the addition of a methyl group to the basic structure of atropine or scopolamine.) These drugs are of particular interest because they pass poorly from the bloodstream into the brain yet they produce characteristic anticholinergic (i.e., antimuscarinic) effects in the peripheral nervous system. Thus, an effect that is produced by scopolamine but is *not* produced by methyl scopolamine can most reasonably be referred to an action of the former on the brain. Conversely, if these two drugs produce comparable effects, then it is most likely that these effects can be referred to peripheral interactions with ACH. (See Carlton, 1963, for an early discussion of the application of this differential to an analysis of the behavioral effects of atropine and scopolamine.)

Chapter 4
Rate-Dependency

IN THE LAST chapter we found that behavioral change can be controlled by at least two factors. These factors are the drug itself and the particular behavior being changed by drug.

We also found that an adequate characterization of a certain drug's action cannot proceed in the absence of dose–response information. Similarly, adequate comparisons of two or more drugs cannot be undertaken in the absence of dose–response data pertinent to the drugs being compared.

However, because behavior is just as important a determinant of changes as is drug itself, it follows that adequate characterization and comparison requires an analysis that extends over a range of behaviors. That is, just as we must study a range of doses, a range of behaviors must also be studied—and this presents a problem.

As noted in Chapter 3, the effects of pentobarbital, for example, vary as a consequence of the behavior being measured (see Figure 3–3). In the example given, behavioral change was imposed on baseline behavior maintained by FI and FR schedules of reinforcement. But how do these baselines differ?

How can FI be compared with FR in a way analogous to the way in which drugs are compared on the basis of dose? Another example will amplify the problem involved: We have seen that DRL schedules (e.g., DRL20) and nondiscriminated avoidance (with RS20) are comparable in that responding in the first instance postpones reinforcement availability, whereas responding in the second postpones shock presentation. But in what way can reinforcement availability be compared to shock absence? How is it possible to say that the absence of a shock of a given intensity is "more" (or "less") than food reinforcement of a given magnitude? The problem is analogous to comparing light and sound: How can we meaningfully say that a given light is "brighter" than a certain sound or that a given sound is "louder" than a certain light?

We can answer these questions by again considering the way different drugs are compared—in terms of dose. For example, 1.0 mg/kg of pentobarbital can be compared with 1.0 mg/kg of amphetamine; 5.0 mg/kg of one drug with 5.0 mg/kg of another drug; and so on. This, of course, is precisely what is done when dose–response curves are constructed.

Dose–response comparisons derive from measurements in a single dimension—dose in mg/kg. For comparison of behavioral baselines another dimension comparable to dose is needed. Such a dimension lies in the fact that all motor behaviors occur at some rate (i.e., number of responses per unit of time). Because all behavioral procedures engender some rate of response, they can be compared on this dimension. For example, the rate engendered by nondiscriminated avoidance could be equal to that engendered by DRL, even though the procedures (reinforcement availability versus shock omission) are not directly comparable. Similarly, the behavior controlled by FI can be compared with that engendered by FR or by any other arrangement that controls rate. We can, then, examine different behaviors in terms of a single dimension: their different rates.

In such comparisons the particulars of different procedures are ignored in the same sense that many of the characteristics of different drugs (e.g., their chemical structure or physical properties) are ignored. In drug comparisons the focus is on dose; in procedure comparisons the focus is on rate. Thus, it is possible to examine the way in which behavioral change varies as a consequence of its characteristic baseline rate, just as drugs can be examined on the basis of dose: When we analyze drugs in terms of dose we are examining a dose-dependency; when we examine behaviors in terms of rate we are examining a rate-dependency.

THE NATURE OF THE DEPENDENCY ON RATE

We know that the behavior being measured can interact with dose to determine drug effect. Let us now consider the prospect that the rate at which this behavior occurs prior to drug administration is the key to characterizing the drug–behavior interaction. If there is indeed a rate-dependency analogous to dose-dependency, what, precisely, is its nature? As we explore the answer to this question we shall begin by considering a single drug, amphetamine, in order to distinguish clearly the several aspects involved.

Behavioral Effects and Baseline Rates   The data in Figure 4–1 have been abstracted from a monumental survey prepared by Dews and Wenger (1977). This survey incorporates virtually all of the then-available data bearing on the behavioral effects of amphetamine; it thus includes an enormous range of procedures (motor activity, various schedules of reinforcement, avoidance procedures, and so on). This array of findings may be categorized in terms of, first, the baseline rates of responding obtained before drug and, second, the dose of amphetamine given. Some of the results obtained from procedures involving the laboratory rat are plotted in the figure.

The upper curve is the dose–response function obtained when the baseline rates of response were low; the lower curve is the analogous function obtained when control rates were high. (The horizontal dashed lines denote the average baseline rates obtained in the absence of drug.) When baseline rates are low, amphetamine increases responding above control levels at low doses but decreases them at very high ones (the point at the far right in the upper graph is below the horizontal line). In contrast, there is a dose-dependent decrease at all doses when baseline rates are high. We can conclude the following:

1. Amphetamine is a stimulant over a range of relatively low doses when baseline rates are low.
2. Amphetamine is a depressant at very high doses even when baseline rates are low.
3. Amphetamine is a depressant over a wide range of doses when baseline rates are high.

Clearly, amphetamine is not simply a depressant or a stimulant. Rather, our conclusions must incorporate a consideration of, first, dose, and second, the relation of drug effect to the baseline rates of responding obtained in the absence of drug. This brings us back to our original question: What is the nature of the dependency of behavioral change on rate?

The data plotted in Figure 4–1 provide an answer, at least for the case of amphetamine. When baseline rates are low, the behavioral change is generally incremental, but when they are high, change is generally decremental. We can, thus, state a rough rule: The effect of amphetamine is inversely related to baseline rate (low baseline rates are increased, high baseline rates are decreased). Given this information, we can refine the rule by looking at rate-dependency in a different way.

Rate-Dependency in Individual Animals   The data in Figure 4–1 were taken from a very large range of procedures; these very different procedures produced different baseline rates, and it is these baseline values, not the procedures themselves, that can predominately determine the effect of drug. Such a compilation of data, however, can produce effects that reflect a statistical average not necessarily characteristic of the individual animal. The question, then, is whether the inverse relation that characterizes rate-dependency holds for the individual animal as well.[1]

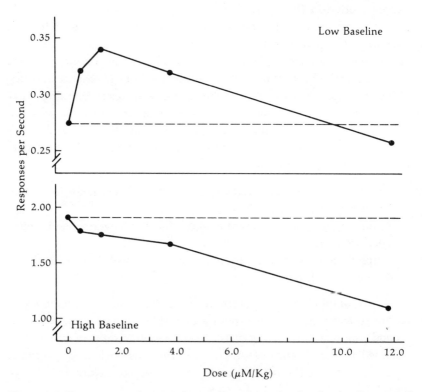

Figure 4–1. Dose–response functions for amphetamine imposed on low baseline rates of responding (top) and on high baseline rates (bottom). (Data from Dews and Wenger, 1977.)

Answering this question requires a way of generating a variety of baseline rates in a single animal in order to determine whether rate-dependency with amphetamine holds (will the low rates increase and the high rates decrease?). The simplest way to obtain a range of baseline rates is to train an animal on a FI schedule. This is true because, as we saw in Chapter 2, rates are very low shortly after reinforcement, but as the interval runs out, rates gradually increase to a high terminal value just prior to the next reinforcement.

Suppose, for example, that an animal has been trained on FI2. We can arbitrarily break each 2-minute interval into six segments of 20 seconds each and then tally the numbers of responses emitted in each segment. Now suppose that the animal emits the sequence of responses shown in row A of Table 4–1; this sequence terminates with reinforcement. The animal then emits a second sequence, shown in row B of Table 4–1. The summed numbers of responses for the two sequences equal the values given in row C; their averages equal those given in row D. Continuation of this process for a large number of intervals will yield a range of stable baseline rates for a single animal.

For amphetamine, the same technique can be applied to the effect of a particular dose so that corresponding sets of values (control versus drug) result. For example, we could obtain averages like those shown in row A of Table 4–2.

Table 4–1

| | Time after reinforcement (sec) | | | | | |
	20	40	60	80	100	120
A. Responses, first sequence	0	2	4	7	15	32
B. Responses, second sequence	4	6	8	13	25	48
C. Total responses	4	8	12	20	40	80
D. Averaged responses	2	4	6	10	20	40

Table 4–2

| | Time after reinforcement (sec) | | | | | |
	20	40	60	80	100	120
A. Averaged responses, post-drug	16	12	12	10	16	20
B. Averaged responses, pre-drug	2	4	6	10	20	40
C. Ratio, post/pre	8.0	3.0	2.0	1.0	0.8	0.5
D. Percent of baseline	800	300	200	100	80	50

The baseline values in row B in Table 4–2 are taken from Table 4–1 (row D). With these two sets of values their ratios can be calculated, as shown in row C; multiplication by 100, yields post-drug values expressed as a percentage of baseline. Thus, drug increased responding in the first three intervals (when baseline rates were low), had no effect in the 80-second interval (when baseline rate was intermediate; 100% indicates no change), and decreased responding in the terminal two intervals (when the baseline was high).

Graphic representation of these data reveals yet another important relationship, as Figure 4–2 makes clear. The values plotted in Figure 4–2A are taken directly from Table 4–2 (rows B and D). As Figure 4–2B indicates, a plot of these same values on logarithmic coordinates results in a simpler, linear relationship.

We have thus far been considering manufactured data. What happens, then, with a real animal given amphetamine? One example, typical of many, is given in Figure 4–3. The rate-dependency is clear.[2] Low control rates are correlated with large relative increases in responding following amphetamine (the values to the upper left of the figure are above the horizontal dashed line, indicating 100%); high control rates are correlated with relative reductions in responding (the values to the lower right are below 100%). Again, when these values are plotted on logarithmic coordinates, as they are in Figure 4–3, a linear relationship of baseline rate and drug effect is obvious.

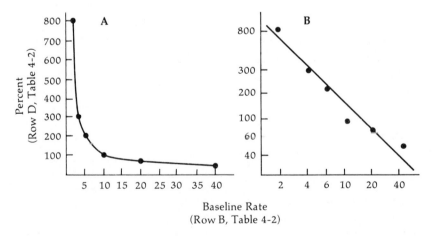

Figure 4–2. Hypothetical rate-dependency functions plotted on linear coordinates *(A)* and logarithmically *(B)*. The plotted values are from rows B and D of Table 4–2.

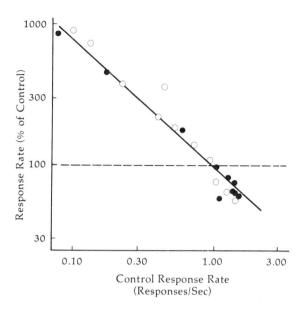

Figure 4–3. Rate-dependency function for a single animal given a single dose of amphetamine. The animal was a monkey that had been trained on an FI schedule of 10 minutes. The open and filled circles are from two separate experiments. (Modified from Kelleher and Morse, 1968, as presented in Pickens, 1977.)

RATE-DEPENDENCY INTERACTIONS

The data in Figure 4–3 were obtained following a single dose of drug. The figure clearly demonstrates a rate-dependency, but we know that behavioral effect is dose-dependent as well as rate-dependent. How, then, does rate-dependency interact with dose-dependency? We shall explore this relationship for two different drugs, amphetamine and chlordiazepoxide.

AMPHETAMINE

Interactions with Dose The data in Figure 4–4 were obtained from groups of rats that were first trained on various schedules of reinforcement and then given different doses of amphetamine. (The schedules are coded in the upper right-hand panel.) The different schedules generated different baseline rates; these control values are plotted on the abscissas of the five graphs. The percentages of increase in responding due to amphetamine are plotted against the ordinates. Note that the coordinates are logarithmic and that each dose produces a linear plot.

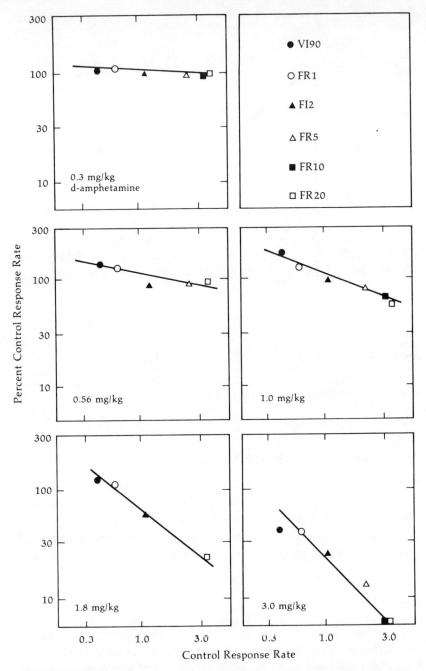

Figure 4–4. Rate-dependency functions for different doses of amphetamine imposed on different baseline rates of responding. The different baselines were generated by the various schedules of reinforcement coded in the upper right panel. (From Heffner, Drawbaugh, and Zigmond, 1974.)

There is a clear rate-dependency at all doses greater than 0.3 mg/kg. Furthermore, the slopes characterizing the rate-dependency become steeper with increasing dose, and each line is displaced downward. Compare, for example, the rate-dependency obtained following 1.0 mg/kg amphetamine with that obtained following 3.0 mg/kg (the middle and lower panels at the right). The line for 3.0 mg/kg is shifted downward and is steeper than that for 1.0 mg/kg. Imagine a point on each line that is centered over the 1.0 value on the abscissa; increasing dose has the effect of shifting the point to lower percentages as well as of rotating the line in a clockwise direction (i.e., steepening its slope).

In effect, the interaction of rate-dependency with dose is such that increasing dose "sharpens" the rate-dependency. Figure 4–4 provides another important implication: Note that the linear relationship that defines rate-dependency holds for all of the schedules studied. This consistency suggests that it is the control rate generated by the schedule that determines the dependency, not the particulars of the schedule itself. Let us now explore this possibility, as well as its limits.

Interactions with Procedure   The cumulative records in Figure 4–5 were produced by different animals trained on different schedules of reinforcement. In particular, rat S21 was trained on FR20 (top), rat S13 on FI2 minutes (middle), and rat S9 on VI90 seconds (bottom). Each generates typical cumulative records (see Chapter 2), and each is responsive to amphetamine. (Note that the recording pen was reset to the baseline after 500 responses had been cumulated.)

As we have already noted, however, the effect of drug interacts with baseline behavior so that very different effects can be obtained. Let us examine the effect of 1.0 mg/kg: Rat S21 (FR20) under control conditions emitted over 2000 responses but emitted less than 1500 following 1.0 mg/kg of drug. In contrast, rat S13 (FI2) was essentially unaffected by this dose, whereas the responding of S9 (VI90) was increased. Furthermore, the overall pattern of results obviously conforms to the pattern to be expected on the basis of rate-dependency: High control rates (FR) are more likely to show a dose-dependent decrease; low control rates (VI) show an increase at low doses followed by a decrease at higher doses; and intermediate rates (FI) are relatively unaffected. This array of relationships could be taken to mean that it is the baseline rate, rather than the particular schedule, that controls the dose–response effect of amphetamine. That is, it might be supposed that the rate that the sched-

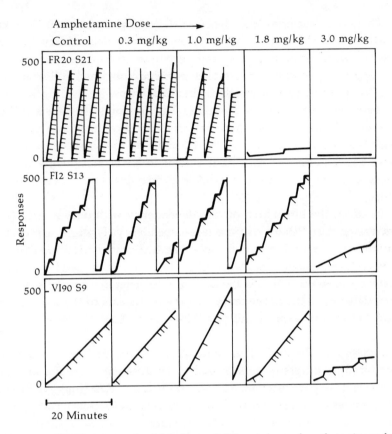

Figure 4–5. Cumulative records of the effects of different doses of amphetamine on behaviors maintained by FR (top), FI (middle), and VI (bottom) schedules of reinforcement. (From Heffner, Drawbaugh, and Zigmond, 1974.)

ule happens to engender is the controlling factor, not the fact that reinforcements are available on the basis of different contingencies.[3]

One way of examining this possibility is to compare two animals that have been exposed to the same schedule. If the animals do differ with respect to their control rates and drug effect differs, then it must be baseline rate that matters. The data in Table 4–3 bear on this prospect. These data reflect the numbers of responses emitted by two animals following various doses of amphetamine; these values are expressed as a percentage of control responding. Both rats had been trained on the same schedule of reinforcement (FR20) but had developed different control rates. In particular, the control rate for Rat 1 was 2.03 responses per second, whereas that for Rat 2 was 5.26 responses per second. Thus, the animal with the lower control rate showed a dose-dependent increase followed by a decrease, whereas the animal with the higher control rate showed only a dose-dependent decrease.

Both animals had been exposed to the same schedule, yet each responded differently to the same doses of amphetamine. Furthermore, this difference was systematically related to baseline rate. Therefore, under some conditions at least, baseline rate—not schedule itself—controls the effect of amphetamine.

How general is this conclusion about amphetamine? Consider yet another set of techniques, the punishment procedures discussed in Chapter 2. The effect of punishment is to suppress ongoing behavior—to produce very low rates of responding. Thus, amphetamine would be expected to increase these low rates if, first, baseline rate controls amphetamine effect in a way that is, second, independent of procedure. But it does not. As we shall see in Chapters 10 and 12, there is no consistent support for the expectation that amphetamine increases the low baseline rates engendered by punishment.

We can put these findings together and conclude the following:

1. A particular procedure can engender a particular baseline rate.
2. This baseline may, in turn, be the primary determinant of the effect of amphetamine (rate-dependency).
3. On the other hand, other procedures (e.g., punishment) can introduce factors that completely override such rate-dependency.

Thus, at a more general level, baseline rate can be a vitally important factor in determining response to drug, but it alone cannot account for all variations in drug response. We shall return to this theme in the following section.

Table 4–3

Dose	Rat 1 (low baseline)	Rat 2 (high baseline)
0.30	114	101
0.56	120	84
1.00	81	39
1.80	53	0
3.00	0	0

Values estimated from Heffner, et.al. 1974.

CHLORDIAZEPOXIDE

Does rate-dependency apply to the effects of drugs other than amphetamine? Let us explore the effects of another drug: chlordiazepoxide, CDZP (see Chapter 12).

The data in Figure 4–6 describe the effects of two doses of CDZP on two classes of behavior. One of these classes was maintained by a schedule of reinforcement that did not involve punishment (panels *B* and *D*); the second schedule did involve punishment and therefore produced relatively lower control rates of responding (panels *A* and *C*).

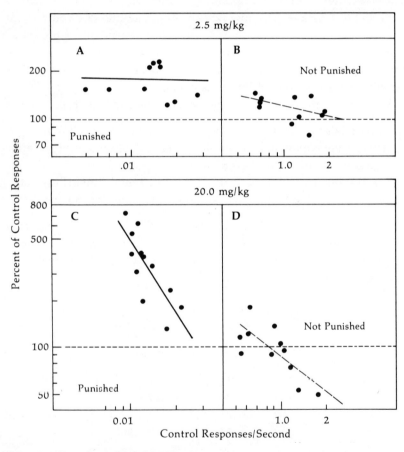

Figure 4–6. Rate-dependency functions for two different doses of chlordiazepoxide (2.5 mg/kg and 20.0 mg/kg) on punished responding (panels *A* and *C*) and on unpunished responding (panels *B* and *D*). (Modified from Cook and Sepinwall, 1976.)

Each point plotted in the figure represents the value for a single animal; each animal was exposed to the punishment and no-punishment contingencies. (See Chapter 12 for procedural details.)

We can begin to examine these data by considering the effects of the higher dose of CDZP (20.0 mg/kg; panels C and D in Figure 4–6. It is clear that, with the usual logarithmic plot, CDZP produces rate-dependent effects. Note, however, that the slopes of the lines describing this dependency are not equal. The dependency is, in effect, "sharpened" by the use of a punishment procedure to generate low control rates (panel C versus D). Thus, as already noted, the details of procedures introduce additional factors that interact with rate-dependency. If control rate were the only factor that differentiated the procedures, a single line would describe all of the data. This is not the case, however.

Now consider the effects of the lower dose (2.5 mg/kg) on unpunished responding (panel B). Again, there is a rate-dependency, but the line describing this dependency is shifted upward and has a less steep slope than that of the line for the 20.0 mg/kg dose (panel D). These dose-dependent relationships thus parallel those for amphetamine (see Figure 4–4).

On the other hand, doses of CDZP increase punished responding, (panels A and C); this is an effect that can not be consistently obtained with amphetamine, as we shall see later. Furthermore, the low dose of CDZP (panel A) produces an increase in responding that is rate-*in*dependent. (The horizontal solid line indicates that there was an increase in responding of about 200% regardless of the control rates characteristic of different animals).

This rather complex array of findings makes a general point that is far more important than the details of the array itself. The point is that three factors—drug, dose of drug, and the baseline rate of responding upon which drug is imposed—can all interact to determine behavioral outcome. Amphetamine and CDZP have qualitatively similar effects on unpunished responding (although amphetamine is more potent); their effects are very different in situations involving punishment; rate-dependency holds in some, but certainly not all, circumstances. Bear in mind, however, that the fact that rate-dependency is not universally applicable does not imply that it can ever be ignored in the analysis of drug action. Let us now consider some of the implications of this fact.

IMPLICATIONS OF INTERACTION

One of the major issues of concern in later chapters has to do with the problem of classifying drugs in terms of their behavioral effects. We want to be able to examine one drug and assign it to one class, examine a second drug and assign it to a different class, and so on. But, when we say that a drug belongs in Class A, for example, we are also saying that it does not belong in Class B. The process of classification thus involves determining specificity of action.

Specificity and Procedural Differences   As we have seen, it is not possible to determine specificity by studying a single dose of a drug. Dose-dependency means that one drug cannot be meaningfully differentiated from another drug on the basis of single-dose comparisons. Identical considerations apply to rate-dependency. The following example illustrates the point.

Suppose an animal is trained to respond for food on a variable interval schedule that generates a relatively high response rate. Now suppose another animal trained on a nondiscriminated avoidance schedule that generates a low overall rate. Once the performance of these animals has stabilized, a drug can be administered over a range of doses, so that the data shown in Table 4–4 are obtained. Given the different drug effects shown at the right of the table, we might conclude that the drug has a specificity of action based on the kinds of reinforcement involved (VI, food; avoidance, shock). We might go on to decide, as others have in analogous circumstances, that the drug is a depressant that increases "fear." That is, the general effect is to decrease responding (VI) over a range of doses, but in a situation involving shock, responding is increased because "fear" is increased; because "fear" is increased, avoidance responding is increased.[4]

Such an interpretation not only incorporates an untested assumption

Table 4–4

Procedure	Control rate	Dose-dependent effect of drug
VI	High	Decrease
Nondiscriminated avoidance	Low	Increase

about the role of "fear" but also totally ignores the possibility of rate-dependency. Might it not be that the apparent procedural specificity (decrease versus increase) lies in the different control rates that the procedures happen to produce? The data we have already considered indicate that this could very well be the case. How, then, can we evaluate the prospect?

We can, first, examine the data for rate-dependency by plotting control rate against drug effect (see Figure 4–4 as an example). Alternatively, we can examine the role of control rate by explicitly varying it. The value of the VI, for example, can be changed to produce control rates comparable to those obtained in the nondiscriminated avoidance situation, as shown in Table 4–5. Such an array of results suggests that the differentiation of drug action on the basis of procedure is not due to kind of reinforcement (food versus shock), to schedule (VI versus avoidance), or to motivational state ("no fear" versus "fear"). Rather, rate-dependency can be assumed to be a primary determining factor of the different drug effects shown in Table 4–4.

Of course, different effects of drug in VI and avoidance responding can be obtained even when baseline rates are matched. With such results, we could then begin to analyse the basis of the difference. But we certainly could not legitimately do so if the role of rate-dependency were not first ruled out.

Is this issue only a hypothetical one based on manufactured data? The following examples show clearly that it is not.

Specificity and Differences in Strains and Species A commonly used technique in behavioral pharmacology involves comparisons of genetically different strains of animals—usually mice because of the availability of a variety of highly inbred strains of this species. Why might we want to compare different strains? One of the major reasons is that such studies can provide a powerful analytic tool for determining the physiologic mechanisms underlying drug action.

For example, suppose we suspect that, of the myriad of physiologic effects a drug may have, one of them controls a particular behavioral effect. Further suppose that we suspect that this one action is due to the drug's interaction with a known endogenous chemical, call it X, in the animal's brain. How might we evaluate the validity of these suspicions? One way would be to select certain strains of animals on the basis of the genetically determined differences in the levels of X in their brains.

Table 4-5

Procedure	Control rate	Dose-dependent effect of drug
VI	Low	Increase
Nondiscriminated avoidance	Low	Increase

Data from one portion of a series of experiments of this kind illustrate the kinds of complications that can arise when rate-dependency is not considered: The experiment involved two strains of mice that differed with respect to the activity of X in the brain; we shall call these strains HX (high activity) and LX (low activity). Different doses of a particular drug were administered to these two groups, and three measures of behavior were recorded. For purposes of illustration, let us consider only the results obtained with a single dose of the drug—the one producing maximal effects.

The values itemized in Table 4-6 indicate the levels of performance recorded following either drug or a control injection of saline.[5] The nature of the activity of X leads to the expectation that drug will produce greater effects in the HX strain than in the LX. The results indicate that this effect was obtained with two of the measures (I and II) but not with the third; compare (a) with (b), (c) with (d), and (e) with (f). In general, the results support expectation—or do they?

Consider the control levels of behavior obtained following saline administration. There is a constant tendency for low control values to be increased by drug and for relatively high values to be decreased. The prospect of rate-dependency rears its head.

The possible role of rate-dependency can be evaluated by computation of the ratio of the rates following drug administration (R) to rates

Table 4-6

Measure	Strain	Saline	Drug
I	HX	0.87	(a) 2.93
	LX	4.93	(b) 1.67
II	HX	1.73	(c) 2.07
	LX	2.27	(d) 0.93
III	HX	1.13	(e) 1.27
	LX	1.80	(f) 1.60

obtained under control conditions (r). These ratios (R/r), derived from Table 4–6, are shown in Table 4–7.

We can, as usual, plot the values of R/r on logarithmic coordinates against the corresponding values of r to obtain the graph shown in Figure 4–7. Note that this graph involves several transformations of the original data in Table 4–6. The following step-by-step consideration describes how the figure was prepared: Consider the original values for Measure I in HX animals (Table 4–6). These values are 0.87 (baseline, r) and 2.93 (rate after drug, R). Thus, $R/r = 2.93/0.87 = 3.37$. This value is shown at (g) in Table 4–7 and is plotted at the upper left in Figure 4–7. Similarly, the values for Measure I in LX animals are 4.93 (r) and 1.67 (R). The value of R/r is 0.34—that is, 1.67/4.93 as shown at (h) in Table 4–7; it is plotted at the lower right of the figure.It is clear that the control levels of responding differ among strains and that these control levels can determine drug effect. What, then, are we to conclude about the possible interaction of X with drug?

On the basis of the data at hand, we cannot conclude anything definitive about the interaction of X and drug.[6] It could be that the baseline levels for the different strains have no relation to X and that, therefore, we are studying rate-dependency but not X itself. On the other hand, we cannot necessarily conclude that X and drug action are totally unrelated. What we need, of course, is a situation in which the baselines of the different strains are matched. If we then obtained differential drug effects we could draw more definitive conclusions about X.[7]

The logic here is the same as that used in our consideration of Tables 4–4 and 4–5, where we were asking a question about specificity of action due to differences in procedure; in this case we are asking about specificity due to strain. Just as we cannot draw clear conclusions without considering dose-dependency, we cannot draw clear conclusions without considering rate-dependency.

Table 4–7

Measure	Strain	r	R/r
I	HX	0.87	(g) 3.37
	LX	4.93	(h) 0.34
II	HX	1.73	1.20
	LX	2.27	0.41
III	HX	1.13	1.12
	LX	1.80	0.89

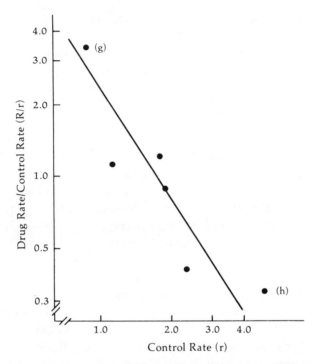

Figure 4–7. Rate-dependency function based on the data presented in Table 4–7. Baseline rates *(r)* are plotted on the abscissa; ratios of post-drug rates to baseline rates *(R/r)* are plotted on the ordinate. The points plotted at the upper left (g) and at the lower right (h) represent the corresponding entries in Table 4–7 (see text for details).

Related considerations apply to comparisons of different species. Comparisons of the behavioral effects of a drug in two species may suggest that one species is affected in a certain way and that the second is affected in another. This conclusion may be correct—but the different species may also have different baselines. Thus, a conclusion about the specificity inherent in different procedures, different strains, or different species must include a consideration of rate-dependency.[8]

Pseudospecificity and "Paradoxical" Effects: MBD   MBD denotes "minimal brain dysfunction," a diagnostic category applied to children characterized by persistent hyperactivity and an accompanying deficit in cognitive performance. Such children typically come to medical attention because their hyperactivity is disruptive and because they often show school performance well below their apparent capabilities.

Amphetamine and related drugs have been widely used to reduce the hyperactivity characteristic of MBD. This reduction in hyperactivity has been generally accepted as being "paradoxical" in that a drug with stimulant effects such as amphetamine decreases behavior. This presumed paradox has, in turn, been used as a diagnostic criterion: If the activity of the child is reduced by amphetamine then, by definition, that child is a victim of MBD.

From our point of view, those conclusions should raise a flag of skepticism. In the first place, the fact that high rates of behavior (hyperactivity) are reduced is not paradoxical; the apparent paradox stems from ignoring the actual behavioral effects of amphetamine and the importance of rate-dependency. Because high rates are commonly reduced by amphetamine, the reduction of activity in certain children can hardly be called "paradoxical," much less "diagnostic." If anything, such an effect is to be expected. It is only when a drug has been simplistically categorized as a stimulant that surprises seem to occur.

If the reduction in activity is not a paradox, however, does this observed action of amphetamine reflect a "dysfunction" at all? It does not seem likely that this is the case: a report by Rapoport and coworkers (1978) shows clearly that amphetamine also reduces activity in children *not* categorized as having MBD. It thus seems more reasonable to assume that children are normally very active and that, as rate-dependency would predict, these normal high rates of responding are reduced by amphetamine.

This is not to say that amphetamine and related drugs may not be useful in the management of certain hyperactive children. Clearly, however, superficial scrutiny of differential drug action can lead to wrong conclusions. In the case of MBD there has been an attempt to classify children on the basis of drug response—to impute a specificity of action that is logically no different from imputing specificity to procedure, strain, or species. When attempts to delineate specificity are undertaken without a consideration of rate-dependency, a psuedospecificity can result. In this instance, it is true that amphetamine and related drugs can decrease motor activity, but this is not paradoxical in itself and certainly does not justify the classification of children as having MBD.

RATE-DEPENDENCY AS EMPIRICAL GENERALIZATION

The basic idea involved in rate-dependency is that behavioral change due to drug is controlled in part by pre-drug rate of responding. At a more particular level, rate-dependency incorporates a feature of this relationship: Low pre-drug rates are likely to increase and high pre-drug rates are likely to decrease as a consequence of drug. At a still more particular level, rate-dependency incorporates a specific quantitative relationship of the kind we have considered.

Why does rate-dependency occur? That is, what mechanisms control it? Why *should* low rates be more likely to increase, and vice versa? These are important questions, but definitive answers remain to be found. As yet there simply are no sufficiently general analyses of behavioral mechanisms that are adequate for an elucidation of the underlying processes that produce rate-dependency. Thus, rate-dependency must be viewed as an empirical generalization—a generalization based on a broad range of experimental evidence. As such, rate-dependency can account for a wide spectrum of drug-induced behavioral phenomena. But it certainly cannot account for all of them, as we have seen and as we shall see again. This does not mean, however, that the possible contribution of rate-dependency can ever be ignored in any sensible analysis of drug action.

Another way of looking at rate-dependency is to view it as a characteristic of the way in which behavioral change is measured. Suppose, for example, that we measure the temperature of a room with a thermometer. Further suppose that we can heat or cool the room by turning on either a furnace or air conditioner. Finally, suppose that the temperature outside the room is 70°F, as measured by another thermometer. We could turn on the furnace and heat the room to 80°. We could then turn off the furnace and open the windows of our room. We would observe, of course, a drop in temperature from a baseline of 80° to 70°. Or we could turn on the air conditioner and cool the room to 60°. If we then turned off the air conditioner and opened the windows, we would observe a shift from a baseline of 60° to 70°.

This example, despite the apparently pointless (and costly) activities involved, does provide a useful metaphor. First, we cannot think of our measurement of room temperature in absolute terms; the changes observed make sense only if our measurement is viewed as part of a system of relative temperatures. Second, a *single* operation (opening the windows) produces *different* effects that vary in relation to the state of the system (with a low initial baseline, temperature will rise; with a high baseline, temperature will drop).

The same kind of relativity characterizes many instances of behavioral change due to drug. The single operation of giving a drug at a single dose (analogous to opening the windows) can either increase or decrease behavior as we measure it (analogous to reading the thermometer in the room). These different effects (increase or decrease) occur in relation to the baseline state of the system upon which the operation is imposed. Moreover, the initial state of the system is reflected in the baseline measure recorded.

Thus, the particular behavior being measured should be considered as a part of a potentially unstable system in which an intervention such as drug will produce effects that are at least partly determined by the initial state of that system. Rate-dependency is no more than an explicit statement about this property of behavioral measurement.[9]

NOTES

1. Sidman (1960) has provided an excellent discussion of the disparity that can occur between statistical averages derived from several individuals and the values for each of these individuals considered alone. As it turns out, averages may not accurately reflect the values characteristic of any of the individuals making up the composite.
2. Rate-dependency is a shift toward a common value in that initially high rates drop and initially low ones increase following drug. This "homogenization" of rates has recently been discussed by Ksir (1981).
3. Sanger and Blackman (1981) have shown that rate-dependency is not due to the different reinforcement densities that can occur with different schedules.
4. As we shall see in later chapters, the invocation of hypothetical states such as "fear" and "anxiety" is not a particularly useful way to analyze the behavioral effects of drugs.
5. The data discussed here are taken from an interesting article by van Abeelen (1974) and have been converted to rates (activity counts per minute). Because we are focusing on only an isolated aspect of his experiments, their overall significance has been substantially distorted.
6. Wenger (1979) has provided a parallel description of the consequences of failing to account for rate-dependency in the analysis of amphetamine effects.
7. In order to evaluate the effect of baseline rate, we need some way to vary that rate just as we did in analyzing the hypothetical data in Tables 4–4 and 4–5. Unfortunately, this cannot be easily done with a measure like motor activity because baseline rate is not under the direct control of the experimenter in a way comparable to the control afforded by the schedules of reinforcement. This limitation also ap-

plies to a measure based on direct observation like those we considered in Chapter 2; there is no simple way to intervene in order to vary the baselines that may, as we have seen, largely determine drug effect.

8. Identical considerations apply to comparisons involving animals of different ages. For example, the drug response in young animals might differ from that in older ones, not because of a difference in biochemical makeup but because of differences in baseline due to age. A failure to consider rate-dependency in this context can lead to fully unwarranted conclusions about differential drug effects and their physiologic bases (see the following discussion of MBD).

9. Despite the potential significance of baseline rate in determining drug effect, such baselines are not uniformly reported in the experimental literature. As a result, some experimental reports are essentially uninterpretable.

Section 2
Drugs as Stimuli

CERTAIN DRUGS ARE known to produce effects that can be consciously felt. Alcohol is one such drug; most people report an awareness of its effects following consumption of even small quantities. In this regard, alcohol is a stimulus, although drugs are not ordinarily thought of as such. As we shall see, however, the concept of drugs as stimuli has two especially useful consequences: It provides a convenient way of organizing a large amount of information; much more important, it generates insights into drug action that would otherwise not be available.

Let us now briefly consider two general features of all stimuli. First, a stimulus is an event that engenders a behavioral change. Indeed, it is the fact of behavioral change that defines the stimulus. That is, although its physical properties can be described, the functional significance of a stimulus can be inferred only from its behavioral consequences. A light, for example, can be described in terms of its intensity and hue, but these physical properties have meaning only because the organism responds to them. The light is not a stimulus for a blind animal; its hue is not a stimulus for a color-blind animal. Similarly, a verbal report of how a person feels following consumption of an alcoholic drink is different from a report that would be given if alcohol had not been consumed.

A second feature of stimuli is that they have multiple properties. Responses to an illuminated electric light bulb could include descriptions of its intensity and hue, as well as of the heat that it generates. Each of these properties can be varied independently, and each can control a different behavior (i.e., a different description).

Let us now turn to a consideration of how these two features—the control of behavior and the multiple properties of stimuli—can be brought together. For our purposes, we can focus on three stimulus characteristics, each of which has figured in previous discussions.

First, a stimulus can have a *cue function*. The discussion of discriminated avoidance in Chapter 2, for instance, described a warning signal that precedes electric shock. Because such a signal can come to control a particular kind of behavior (avoidance), we know that the stimulus has acted as a cue for the animal. Second, certain kinds of stimuli have an *aversive function;* the electric shock used in avoidance and punishment procedures is a case in point. Finally, other stimuli, like food and water, can come to control approach behavior. Such stimuli have a positive *reinforcing function.*

We shall consider each of these three characteristics in the chapters that lie ahead. As we do so, a familiar theme will emerge: behavioral effects can vary as a consequence of an overall system in which stimuli are only one part.

A useful analogy for this kind of complexity can be found by again referring to the illuminated light bulb: a nocturnal animal such as the rat may avoid the stimulus because of its brightness; if the ambient temperature is low, however, the rat may approach the bulb for its heat. As we shall see, drugs are also stimuli, and their effects are comparably complex.

Chapter 5
Reinforcement Functions

AS JUST NOTED, certain stimuli, like food or water, can act as reinforcements when they are presented. These stimuli are called reinforcers to the extent that they maintain the behavior upon which their presentation is contingent. Although these stimuli most certainly control consummatory behavior, the experimenter merely arranges the presentation of the stimulus; the animal does the rest. Thus, from the point of view of the experimenter, presentation of food, say, is operationally the same as turning on a light when the animal emits some response. If this arrangement of response and stimulus leads to repetition and maintenance of the response, the animal has learned and the stimulus is a reinforcer. But can drugs also be reinforcing stimuli?

Certain drugs such as nicotine and alcohol do apparently maintain substantial chains of behavior—that is, these drugs seem to have reinforcement functions if the sales of cigarettes and of alcoholic beverages are used as guides. However, the variables that are involved in smoking and drinking behaviors are vastly complex. (Recall that amphetamine seems to be a stimulant—it is in some cases and it is not in others.) Clearly, generalizations based on casual observation can lead to erroneous conclusions, as they have in other contexts. With this consideration, let us proceed to relatively simple situations in which the relevant variables can be isolated and analyzed.

Are some drugs reinforcers, and are there some drugs that are not?

Moreover, how can we find out? Answering these questions requires a procedure in which some behavior is made contingent on drug ingestion in the way that it is with food and water. If the drug maintains responding, as food or water will, then the drug is indeed a reinforcing stimulus.

Unfortunately, animals will not ordinarily consume drugs as they will food or water, presumably because many drugs have an aversive (e.g., bitter) taste. The way around this problem is to circumvent the consummatory behavior and to inject the drug directly into the animal. A schematic of an apparatus that can be used to provide such circumvention is shown in Figure 5–1 (compare Figure 2–1). The animal can operate a switch by depressing a lever in the response chamber. This response operates the programming circuitry, which in turn operates an infusion pump that delivers a small, measured amount of drug to the animal via a catheter implanted in its vein. This kind of apparatus provides a means for determining whether an animal will self-inject a drug and thus provide us with information about whether the drug can or cannot act as a reinforcing stimulus.

The data plotted in Figure 5–2 are from an early report using this procedure (Deneau, Yanagita, and Seevers, 1969). In this study a monkey was allowed to self-inject morphine over the course of 26 weeks; the stable level of self-dosing (about 75 mg/kg/day) is shown in the top panel of the figure. The daily cycles of self-injection during week 5 and

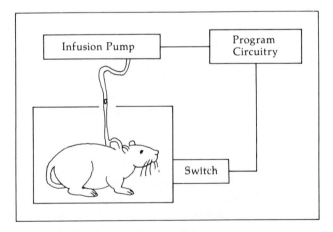

Figure   5–1. Schematic   representation   of   an   apparatus   for   studying   the self-administration of drugs in laboratory animals; compare Figure 2–1. (Redrawn from Pickens, 1977.)

week 26 are shown in the other two panels. Clearly, the opportunity to self-administer morphine maintains reliable and stable patterns of behavior.

Figure 5–3 provides a comparison of responding maintained by two reinforcing stimuli, food and injections of the drug cocaine, as studied by Tessel and Woods (1975). In this experiment, a monkey could obtain food pellets on a FR30 schedule when a red light was on, and it could obtain 30.0 μg/kg injections of cocaine when a white light was on. Apart from the initial burst of responding immediately following the first transition from food to cocaine, it is clear that, first, both stimuli

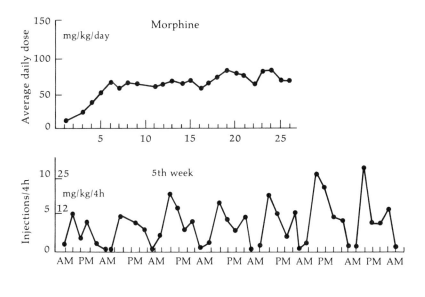

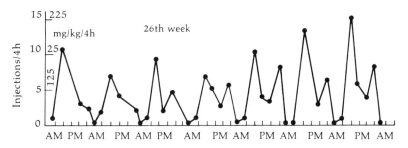

Figure 5–2. Patterns of self-administration for a single monkey. The total daily amounts of morphine administered over the course of 26 weeks are shown at the top; the cycles of self-administration within successive days of week 5 (middle) and week 26 (bottom) are also shown. (From Deneau, Yanagita, and Seevers, 1969.)

maintain comparable behaviors, and second, both patterns of behavior are characteristic of FR schedules. Cocaine, like food, is a reinforcing stimulus.

Applications of this technique to a variety of other drugs permit them to be classified in terms of whether or not they have been shown to maintain self-administration in monkeys. A partial listing is presented in Table 5–1.[1] The drugs in the first grouping have been shown to maintain self-administration, although the data for a few (those indicated by the asterisks) are somewhat contradictory. This listing includes drugs that produce clear physical dependence (the opiates) as well as those that are known to be "abused": alcohol, the amphetamines, the barbitu-

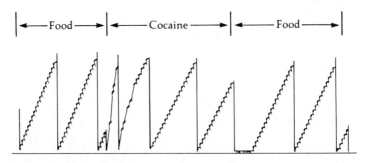

Figure 5–3. Cumulative records of responding maintained by food or by cocaine self-administration. (Modified from Tessel and Woods, 1975.)

Table 5–1

Drugs that are self-administered	Drugs that do not maintain self-administration
1. Alcohol	11. Imipramine
2. Amphetamine and related drugs	12. Mescaline
	13. Phenothiazines
3. Barbiturates	14. Scopolamine
4. Caffeine*	
5. Cocaine	
6. Nicotine*	
7. Opiates (morphine and related drugs)	
8. Procaine	
9. Phencyclidine (PCP)	
10. THC (active component in marijuana)*	

rates and cocaine, phencyclidine, and THC. (Note that the group includes stimulants, depressants, and some drugs that are not clearly either.) The list also includes drugs that fall into neither category: caffeine, nicotine, and procaine. Thus, all drugs that are addicting or "abused" may be reinforcing, but not all drugs that are reinforcing are necessarily either. We shall return to some of the implications of this fact later in the chapter.

The drugs in the second grouping do not seem to maintain self-administration in laboratory animals. The listing includes an anticholinergic (scopolamine), an antidepressant (imipramine; see Chapter 14), and several phenothiazines of the kind discussed in Chapter 13. More to the point, none of these drugs has been shown to be voluntarily self-administered by humans,[2] whereas those in the first grouping generally are. There is, therefore, a general correspondence between the laboratory demonstration of reinforcing function and voluntary intake by humans.

Note, however, that the first listing includes procaine, a local anesthetic chemically related to cocaine. Although procaine is demonstrably reinforcing, it is not known to be self-administered by humans. On the other hand, mescaline is a hallucinogen that *is* self-administered by humans but has not been shown to be reinforcing in the laboratory. There are, then, exceptions to the correspondence of self-administration in the laboratory and in humans.

FALSE POSITIVES AND FALSE NEGATIVES

Exceptions to the correspondence of two measures are, for our purposes, of greater general significance than whether certain drugs are or are not reinforcing stimuli. Whenever two measures are considered, a question arises about the extent to which the categorization provided by one measure corresponds to that provided by the other. In the case at hand, self-administration in humans can be regarded as the criterion measure. The question thus becomes one about the extent to which our laboratory measure (self-administration in animals) predicts the criterion. In order to answer this question, the drugs in Table 5–1 can be categorized in a different format, shown in Table 5–2.

The numbers in Table 5–2 denote the drugs listed in Table 5–1. Our criterion of self-administration in humans is thus predicted reasonably well by our laboratory measure. That is, "yes" to the question about reinforcing function in the laboratory usually corresponds to "yes" to the criterion question (self-administered in humans).

Table 5–2

Self-administered by humans?	Reinforcing in the Laboratory?	
	No	*Yes*
Yes	(A) 12 (False negative)	(B) 1, 2, 3, 4, 5, 6, 7, 9, 10 (True positives)
No	(C) 11, 13, 14 (True negatives)	(D) 8 (False positives)

The entries at (B) represent **true positives:** That is, the laboratory response is "positive" (the drugs are reinforcing), and this is also "true" for our criterion. In other words, both measures generate "yes" indicators.

The entries at (C) are **true negatives.** In this case, the three drugs have not been shown to be reinforcing in the laboratory, and they are not known to be self-administered by humans (see, however, the following discussion). Thus, the answers to both questions are "No," and there is therefore a correspondence between measures.

The entry at (A) is a **false negative.** It has not been shown to be reinforcing; therefore, it would not be expected to be self-administered by humans—but this expectation is false. The entry at (D) is a **false positive:** It *is* demonstrably reinforcing in the laboratory and therefore, would be expected to be self-administered by humans, but this expectation is also false. In both instances, laboratory procedure gives rise to an expectation (positive or negative) that is not borne out by the criterion.

LIMITATIONS IN INTERPRETATION OF RESULTS

It should not be surprising that a laboratory procedure can generate false positives and false negatives. In fact, it is more surprising that the correlation of the laboratory data and self-administration in humans is as good as the data indicate. After all, our example involves rats and monkeys self-administering drugs under artificial conditions versus voluntary intake by humans in extraordinarily complex psychologic and social circumstances. Indeed, our criterion can be correctly met in 12 of 14 cases (86%). This surely means that the fact that a drug is a reinforcing stimulus has an important bearing on whether it will be self-administered by humans. However, our approach to how this relationship should be interpreted must be cautious, because such interpretation must consider two severe limitations on the kinds of data just discussed.

The Uncertainty of "No"   Any statement that a phenomenon does not occur immediately presents the problem of confirming a universal negative. That is, if we conclude that something does not occur, we cannot also conclude that it will never occur. We can say that a phenomenon has not been demonstrated, but this does not mean that it may not be at some future time—we can say "No," but we must never say "Never".

These considerations are obviously pertinent to the entries in Table 5–2. For example, mescaline has not been shown to be reinforcing in laboratory animals. But it is not certain whether this fact is truly characteristic of the drug or whether the laboratory techniques actually used were merely inadequate to the demonstration. Similarly, we can conclude that some drugs are not self-administered by humans, but we cannot be certain that the data are complete—that is, it may be that they *are* self-administered but that the fact has simply not been reported. In this light, the entry at (D), for procaine, may be truly a false positive, or it may only appear that procaine is not self-administered by humans because a sufficient number of people have thus far failed to try it.

Because we can never say "Never," three of the four groupings in Table 5–2 necessarily represent tentative conclusions: We can be confident only in the single instance of true positives, the groupings labeled (B) in the table. This is so because it is only in this instance that we can say "Yes" with respect to both laboratory data and human self-administration. Thus, interpretation of relationships like those in Table 5–2 must be cautious ones.

Failure of Inclusion   A second limitation inherent in our example is that the study has not included a variety of prescription and non-prescription drugs that are actually consumed.

The pharmaceutical industry is a large and prosperous one because both the variety and the quantity of drugs self-administered by humans are enormous. Some of these are taken in response to "doctor's orders" (see Note 2); still others (e.g., aspirin or decongestants) are self-administered without medical directive, presumably because of the symptomatic relief they provide. Vitamins, however, are self-administered in vast quantities that are well beyond established dietary requirements and for which there is no clearly established benefit.

If all of these drugs were to be evaluated in the laboratory, it is certain that not all of them would be found to act as reinforcing stimuli. Thus, the strength of the relationship in Table 5–2 is partly actifactual because the table has failed to include a very large number of drugs that are, in fact, self-administered by humans. Just what conclusions, then, do the data in Table 5–2 permit? Clearly, not all drugs self-administered by humans are demonstrably reinforcing, nor is it necessarily true that drugs *not* been shown to be reinforcing will *not* be self-administered (the uncertainty of "No"). Our only possible legitimate conclusion is that, if a drug has been shown to be a reinforcing stimulus, it is very likely, but not certain to be self-administered by humans.

REINFORCEMENT AND ABUSE

A great deal of interest has been focused on the possible relationship of reinforcement function to the "abuse" of certain drugs by humans. Indeed, if we consider the drugs at (B) in Table 5–2, there is a good correspondence of the two phenomena: Alcohol, the amphetamines, the barbiturates, cocaine, the opiates, and phencyclidine can all be said to have been abused. But, as we shall see, this correspondence is less compelling than it might at first seem.

In evaluating the character of this correspondence, we must consider two issues: first, we must address the question of what is meant by drug "abuse"; second, we must evaluate the detailed nature of the presumed link between reinforcement function and abuse liability.

THE DEFINITION OF "ABUSE"

It is a widely held view that any use of a drug that leads to demonstrable physical or psychologic harm can reasonably be called "abused." As we have noted, most of the drugs at (B) in Table 5–2 meet this definition. However, all of them do not; consider caffeine, nicotine, or THC (the active ingredient in marijuana).

Can caffeine properly be said to be abused? It is certainly self-administered in coffee, tea, and various cola beverages, but does this use lead to demonstrable harm? It could be said, of course, that caffeine will produce demonstrable harm if used in sufficient quantity. But this can be said of any drug. In other words, the fact that a drug has the *potential* for abuse does not mean that it can be labeled as an abused substance.

Next, consider nicotine. It is clear that the smoking of tobacco poses demonstrable health hazards. It is far less certain, however, whether this is a consequence of nicotine itself or whether the danger is due to the various other products of combustion contained in cigarette smoke. Thus, it cannot be said unequivocally that nicotine is an abused substance.[3]

Abuse of THC, the active ingredient in marijuana, is also questionable. The topic of whether smoking marijuana leads to demonstrable harm is an unusually controversial one. It can be said, nonetheless, that the possibility of actual harm due to THC has been far less clearly shown than has the unquestionable harm due to the use of alcohol and of opiates like heroin and morphine.

Are nicotine, THC, and caffeine truly abused substances? The answer is not entirely clear. It *is* clear, however, that the label of "abuse" cannot be applied to these drugs in precisely the same sense that it is to drugs such as the opiates, amphetamines, barbiturates, and alcohol. Thus, the idea that reinforcing drugs also have abuse potential is not as straightforward as it might at first seem. The supposition that reinforcement function predicts abuse liability hinges very much on what is meant by "abuse." It is true that drugs known to be harmful, as they are actually used, are demonstrably reinforcing. On the other hand, all drugs that are reinforcing may not qualify as being abused, at least in the sense that "abuse" implies demonstrable harm. Finally, the fact that a drug has *not* been shown to be reinforcing does not, as we have seen, necessarily mean that it is "safe"—immune to abuse.

REINFORCEMENT FUNCTION AND ABUSED DRUGS

Another aspect of the issue we are discussing has to do with the very imperfect relationship of reinforcement function and drugs that clearly are abused. The opiates, for example, are potent reinforcers (see Figure 5–2), yet relatively few people actually do abuse them. Why, then, should drugs that are so powerfully reinforcing not be more widely used than they are? The answer lies, of course, in the fact that a large number of variables determine whether a drug is or is not self-administered. Such variables include cost, possible criminal prosecution, the accurately perceived potential for physical harm, and a variety of moral and ethical prohibitions.

Again, we see that drugs do not simply and directly modulate behavior; an adequate analysis must include characterization of the behavioral systems in which they do—and do not—produce particular effects.[4] This is not to say that the demonstration that a drug can act as a reinforcing stimulus is an irrelevant bit of information. Such findings alone, however, cannot be used to draw simple conclusions about drug abuse. The demonstration of reinforcing function is only a crucial first step in the analysis of the variables that control human self-administration.[5]

NOTES

1. The data in Table 5–1 represent a somewhat oversimplied summary of material presented by Schuster and Johanson (1981), Johanson (1978), and Griffiths, Brady, and Bradford (1979). The originals should be consulted for details. In addition, some of the complications introduced by limited versus unlimited access to drug have been discussed by Balster and Wolverton (1982).
2. These drugs may, of course, be self-administered because they have been prescribed by a physician. There is no evidence, however, that they are voluntarily taken in the absence of such a directive.
3. The increasing popularity of decaffeinated coffee and of "low tar and nicotine" cigarettes indicate that there is not a direct linkage of self-administration to drug level. The voluntary intake involved in coffee drinking and cigarette smoking is controlled by an array of complex interacting variables, not drug intake in itself.
4. Some of these factors have been discussed in an important article by Schuster, Renault, and Blaine (1979).
5. A recurrent question about self-administration is whether drugs act as "real" reinforcers—that is, whether they act in the same way that food or water act in appropriately deprived animals. This question has been addressed by Johanson (1978); the answer she provides is convincingly affirmative.

Chapter 6

Aversive Functions

THE PROTOTYPE OF an aversive stimulus is electric shock. Animals will escape from it, and given the opportunity, they will avoid it. Alternatively, it can be used to suppress behavior in either punishment or CER situations. Are these properties also characteristic of drugs?[1]

As we shall see, there are two general ways in which drugs can be shown to be aversive stimuli. First, some drugs are demonstrably aversive when administered to animals that have become physically dependent on the opiates. A second approach involves procedures that do not require dependent animals. For this approach we shall consider two experimental paradigms that have been used to demonstrate aversiveness: one involves the self-injection procedures mentioned earlier; another involves injecting animals after they have ingested a food to elicit aversion that is uniquely associated with gustatory stimuli.

AVERSIVENESS IN DEPENDENT ANIMALS: NARCOTIC ANTAGONISTS

An animal that has been chronically dosed with a certain drug can become dependent on that drug. Such dependence has traditionally been called *physical dependence* because when drug administration is terminated, a set of physical withdrawal symptoms occur.

The most notorious drugs of this kind are, of course, the opiates (e.g., heroin). Withdrawal from the opiates can induce the following symptoms: restlessness, chills, hot flashes, lacrimation, intense cramps, vomiting, diarrhea, perspiration, muscle twitches, anorexia, and insomnia. These same symptoms can be precipitated by certain other drugs (the so-called narcotic antagonists) even though the dose of the addicting drug (e.g., the heroin) is maintained. We shall consider two of these antagonists, naloxone and nalorphine.[2]

It is clear that dependent animals will respond to terminate injections of these antagonists. An example is shown in Figure 6–1. In a study by Woods (1978), a morphine-dependent monkey could escape from an infusion of saline or of naloxone by emitting 20 responses (i.e., the schedule was FR20). As the cumulative record at the top of the figure indicates, saline did not maintain this escape behavior. On the other hand, the remaining two records clearly show that the opportunity to escape from naloxone did maintain behavior at both the 0.0003-mg/kg and the 0.001-mg/kg doses. Note that the higher dose maintained more stable levels of responding.

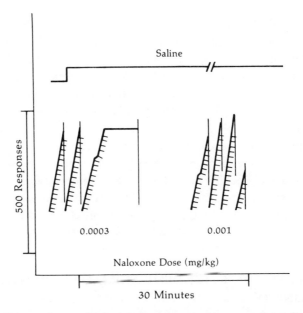

Figure 6–1. Cumulative records of responding maintained by escape from saline or naloxone infusion (0.0003 and 0.001 mg/kg/infusion). The animal was dependent on morphine, and morphine injections were maintained throughout the experiment. (Modified from Woods, 1978.)

Neutral stimuli that are associated only with naloxone infusions can also maintain behavior. That is, animals will respond to terminate a stimulus that is correlated with injection of the antagonist. Thus, these aversive stimuli can confer their aversive properties on another, neutral stimulus. The situation is, therefore, analogous to the one discussed in the context of discriminated avoidance in Chapter 2: That is, a stimulus such as electric shock can maintain escape behavior, and another stimulus associated with it can maintain avoidance behavior.

Conditioned aversions can also be demonstrated in CER paradigms like those discussed in Chapter 2 (Goldberg and Schuster, 1967). In this case, pairing of a neutral simulus with an injection of antagonist (in dependent animals) leads to suppression of responding during the stimulus. This effect is analogous to one that would be obtained were electric shock used in place of the antagonist.[3]

AVERSIVENESS IN NONDEPENDENT ANIMALS

DIRECT INJECTION

The demonstration of aversiveness for the drugs just discussed requires dependent monkeys; their aversiveness inheres in the fact that they are narcotic antagonists. Other drugs appear to be aversive in nondependent animals.

Unfortunately, this area has not been nearly so well explored as has that relating to the prospect that drugs can act as reinforcing stimuli. Injections of the neuroleptic phenothiazines (see Chapter 13) are known, however, to maintain avoidance or escape behavior.

The phenothiazines are among the drugs previously described as having no reinforcing effect (see Table 5–1). Of these drugs, only the phenothiazines have clearly been shown to act as aversive stimuli. Whether the other drugs are truly neutral, or whether techniques adequate to demonstrate their aversiveness have not yet been developed, is not yet known.

As things stand, only the phenothiazines have been shown to be aversive stimuli in situations involving termination of injection by the emission of a particular response; that is, injection is analogous to the electric shocks used in the procedures discussed in Chapter 2. However, use of a different procedure produces different results. As we shall see, the particulars of the behavior being studied once again determine the behavioral effect of drug.

CONDITIONED TASTE AVERSION

Suppose a rat is allowed to eat some food and then is injected with amphetamine; drug follows ingestion. When ingestion of food is permitted a second time but is not followed by drug administration, measurement of food intake shows that the animal eats much less if it eats at all. In such an arrangement, a stimulus (amphetamine) follows a given behavior (ingestion). The marked reduction in the subsequently measured behavior shows amphetamine to be a stimulus that has aversive properties. In particular, the stimuli associated with food have taken on the properties of the aversive stimulus (drug) just as a neutral stimulus can take on aversive properties because of its association with electric shock.

Now suppose that amphetamine is injected after the animal has emitted some other behavior, such as lever pressing. Under these circumstances, an equivalent dose of drug does not suppress behavior. The suppressant effect of drug seems to be peculiar to ingestive behaviors; such suppression is generally referred to as *conditioned taste aversion* because the gustatory stimuli associated with food itself uniquely control aversive behavior. "Aversion" in this context means, however, only that the animal stays away from the food; it therefore eats less than it normally would. Viewed in this way, a conditioned taste aversion is an instance of punishment of an unusual kind.

Amphetamine is not the only drug that can engender aversion. In fact, the suspicion arises that almost any drug, at some dose, can produce this effect. For example, an only partial list of drugs that have been shown to have this property is given in Table 6-1. Several comments on this list are in order: First, the list contains some drugs (e.g., methyl

Table 6-1

Alcohol
Amphetamine
Atropine
Chlordiazepoxide
Formalin
Lithium
Mescaline
Methyl atropine
Methyl scopolamine
Morphine
Scopolamine

scopolamine and methyl atropine) that do not enter from the blood-stream into the brain (see Chapter 3, Note 8). The aversion that they control thus appears to be based on the peripheral effects of drug.

Second, it is true that some of the drugs produce obvious signs of sickness in the animals studied. It has been suggested, therefore, that some sort of conditioned illness is involved. However, aversions can be obtained without the appearance of overt signs of sickness due to drug. Although the animal may be ill in some way that cannot be observed, it is useless to debate the possibility because we can never know any-thing more than the fact that observable signs of illness are not neces-sary.

A third feature is that the degree of aversion can be reduced by prior exposure to either the food or the drug. If the animal is given prior expe-rience with the food (not associated with drug) or with the drug (not associated with food), subsequent association of food with drug will have a substantially reduced effect. Thus, a degree of "novelty" in both classes of stimuli (gustatory cues and drug stimuli) seems to be required.

Furthermore, aversive effects can be obtained even if the interval be-tween ingestion and treatment is measured in *hours.* In contrast, punish-ing effects of stimuli like electric shock can typically be obtained only in the range of a few seconds. Suppose an animal is allowed to eat and then is injected one-half hour after its meal. Now suppose that food is again presented two days later. We will find that intake is markedly reduced. If, on the other hand, an animal is allowed to complete a meal and then is given an electric shock one-half hour later, we will surely not find a reduction in eating. Thus, this demonstration of aversive properties is special in that particular behaviors (ingestion) and unusual temporal parameters are involved. Although these conditions may be special, the facts themselves should not at this point be surprising. We have, after all, repeatedly found that the particulars of the behavior being measured can determine drug effect.

DUALITY OF STIMULUS FUNCTION

We began this chapter by considering naloxone and nalorphine, opiate antagonists that can act as aversive stimuli in opiate-dependent animals. We then considered the phenothiazines, a group of drugs with aversive functions that have been demonstrated with self-injection procedures. Finally, we saw that a number of drugs can form the basis of taste aver-sions (see Table 6–1).

It turns out that some of the drugs in this last category can also be shown to be reinforcing stimuli (Chapter 5). To make matters still more complex, it can also be shown that naloxone and nalorphine are self-administered by *non* dependent animals; these drugs, aversive in dependent animals, are otherwise reinforcing stimuli (see Woods, 1978).

We are thus confronted with a complex array of phenomena: a drug can be either reinforcing or aversive. Some of the relevant comparisons are given in Table 6–2. As summarized in the table, alcohol, amphetamine, and morphine (a) are reinforcing in that they maintain self-administration, yet they are aversive in that they can form the basis of taste aversions; nalorphine and naloxone (b) are reinforcing in nondependent animals but aversive in dependent ones; mescaline and scopolamine (c) have not been shown to be reinforcing with self-administration procedures but are active in taste aversion paradigms; only the phenothiazines conform to "common sense" expectation in that they are not reinforcing with self-injection techniques and can be shown to be aversive.

These data bear on a much more general point. The stimulus properties of drug obviously do not inhere solely in drug itself. Rather, it is clear that a drug may be either reinforcing or aversive as a consequence of the multiplicity of variables that can interact to determine behavioral outcome. The relevant question, then, is not whether a drug is or is not reinforcing or aversive—as if these were mutually exclusive possibilities—but in which circumstances a given drug is one or the other.[4]

This idea is fundamentally no different from the one presented at the beginning of Section II when we considered the different roles an illuminated light bulb might have: It can be aversive, to be sure, but in a cold

Table 6–2

	Development of taste aversions	Drugs shown to be aversive by: Avoidance, escape, or suppression procedures involving self-injection
Self-administered	(a) Alcohol Amphetamine Morphine	(b) Nalorphine* Naloxone*
Not Self-administered	(c) Mescaline Scopolamine	(d) Phenothiazines

*In opiate-dependent monkeys.

environment, it can control approach behavior. Drugs are stimuli; there is therefore no reason to suppose they cannot have the same kind of duality of function.[5] We have also seen that stimuli can have yet another function in that they can serve as cues for differential responding. Because drugs are stimuli, they would be expected to have this property as well as aversive and reinforcing functions. We shall examine that expectation in the following chapter.

NOTES

1. Much of the material discussed here has been described in greater detail by Johanson (1978).
2. Naloxone and nalorphine block opiate receptors but are themselves largely devoid of biologic effect. They thus abruptly precipitate the withdrawal symptoms that would occur if the opiate were actually discontinued (see Chapter 3).
3. It is of particular interest that the animals showed some withdrawal symptoms during the stimulus itself; that is, there was a "conditioned withdrawal" that occurred even though opiate administration was maintained and the antagonist was not given.
4. A striking example of such duality of stimulus function can be found in the effects of electric shock. Shock is, of course, the prototypical aversive stimulus. Yet, under some circumstances, shock can serve as a reinforcing stimulus that will *maintain* responding much the same way that food and water can. Data of this kind, and their implications, have been discussed in excellent articles by McKearney (1976) and by Morse, McKearney, and Kelleher (1977).
5. At a still more general level, this discussion of duality of function relates to ideas that emerged at the end of the discussion of rate-dependency. Recall that in that context we developed the idea that the system of variables in which a particular behavior occurred was the determinant of outcome. A parallel conceptualization applies to drug: whether a drug will be aversive or reinforcing, a stimulant or a depressant, depends not on the drug alone but on the behavioral system in which the drug acts.

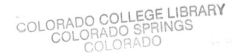

Chapter 7
Cue Functions

WE HAVE THUS far considered drugs as reinforcing and aversive stimuli. Let us now turn to a discussion of their cue functions. The first question is whether drugs can, in fact, serve as cues for differential responding.[1]

Suppose an animal is reinforced for emitting one response —R1—when one stimulus is present and is never reinforced when that stimulus is absent. Suppose a second response—R2—is reinforced only when a second stimulus is present. Under these circumstances the animal will come to emit only R1 in the presence of the first stimulus and only R2 in the presence of the other. The animal will have learned to discriminate the stimuli.

Such discriminations have routinely been obtained and studied for many years. The stimuli in question have, however, traditionally been exteroceptive ones, such as sounds of different frequency or lights of different color. It is only recently that drugs have been studied in this way; as it turns out, animals can make discriminations on the basis of drug condition.[2]

A simple version of this kind of discrimination involves escape learning. An animal can learn to escape from electric shock by making one of two responses. However, only one response—R1—leads to escape when the animal has received a drug (pentobarbital, say); the other response—R2—does not work. The complement holds when the animal has received a control injection of saline; R1 does not provide escape, but R2 does. The data can be treated in terms of relative number of responses that are correct with regard to the prevailing stimulus (drug) conditions. Suppose, for example, the animal is allowed to respond 200 times, 100 when it has received pentobarbital and 100 when it has not. Further suppose that the number of R1 responses following pentobarbital (correct when drug has been given) is 90 and the number of R2 responses (incorrect) is 10, and that, in addition, the number of R2 responses (correct when drug has not been given) is 95 and the number of R1 responses (incorrect) is 5. The percentages of correct responses would thus be 90% and 95%. On the other hand, if the animal were not discriminating at all, R1 and R2 responses would occur by chance; the animal would respond at a 50% level in both conditions. Data of these kinds are shown in Figure 7–1. The data in this figure are from a study by Overton (1964) in which three groups of rats that were required to learn to escape under the conditions summarized in Table 7–1.

In this study, the experimental group was given either drug (D; pentobarbital, 25.0 mg/kg) or no drug (ND; saline) at different times. In contrast, the two control groups were given only one kind of injection (D or ND) before each session. Thus, in the experimental group, correct responses were consistently associated with different drug conditions (R1 with drug; R2 with no drug), whereas the control groups had one correct response to learn (R1 for the D control, R2 for the ND control).

The upper panel in the figure presents the data from the no drug (ND) periods for the experimental group in comparison with the performance of the ND control. It is evident that the experimental animals performed just as well as the control animals that were not required to make the D versus ND discrimination. Both groups of animals learned, and both learned equally well.

The lower panel presents the data from the complementary drug conditions. Again, the experimental group, when drugged, performed just as well as the group that was trained only under the D condition. (The somewhat slower rate of learning in these animals, as compared to that shown in the upper panel, undoubtedly reflects the sedative effects of the drug.)

Put crudely, each animal in the experimental group was behaving as if it were two animals. That is, the discrimination of D from ND was so complete that the animals performed as they would have if no discrimination had been required (as was the case in the control groups).[3]

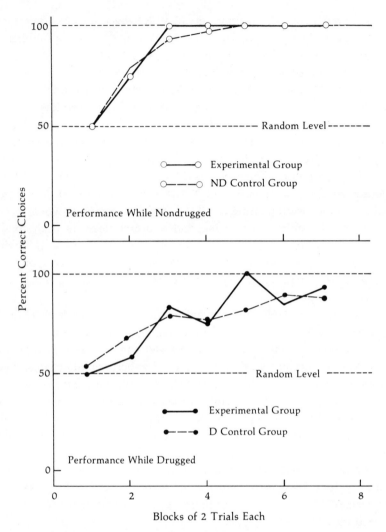

Figure 7–1. Percentages of correct responses when animals had been injected either with saline (top) or with pentobarbital (bottom). Control animals received only one kind of injection (ND or D; "no drug" or "drug"), whereas experimental animals received either on different occasions. (From Overton, 1964.)

Table 7-1

Group	Injection	Correct response
Experimental	D	R1
	ND	R2
D Control	D	R1
ND Control	ND	R2

DIFFERENCES IN DISCRIMINABILITY

The effects described in Figure 7-1 were obtained with only one drug at one dose. Such a limitation naturally leads to a consideration of possible effects with other drugs and at other doses.

DOSE EFFECTS

Variation of the dose of a drug stimulus produces, in effect, variation in its intensity. Analogously, the intensity of a buzzer is related to the "amount" of sound it produces. Thus, a control injection of saline (ND) has, by definition, a zero intensity.

As a general rule, increasing dose increases the extent of the D–ND discrimination obtained in situations like the one used to obtain the data in Figure 7-1. That is, a high dose (analagous to a loud sound) should be more readily discriminated from saline (silence) than is a low dose (analagous to a low intensity sound). This means that it is possible to vary the doses of different drugs and compare them in terms of their overall discriminability. (Such comparisons are, of course, limited by the debilitation that high doses may produce.)

DISCRIMINABILITY OF DIFFERENT DRUGS

Not all drugs are equally discriminable from saline, as Table 7-2 indicates.

As we saw in Figure 7-1, animals can readily learn to discriminate barbiturates (entry 3). In contrast, they learn more slowly with amphetamine (entry 10), for example, and still more slowly with the group of phenothiazines (entry 18). This differential discriminability raises two additional issues.

Relations Among Stimulus Functions   The data in Table 7-2 bear directly on a point discussed in our initial consideration of drugs as a stimuli. A stimulus can have a reinforcing function, it can have an aversive func-

Table 7-2

Readily discriminated	Moderately discriminated	Poorly discriminated
1. Alcohol	10. Amphetamines	16. Lithium
2. Atropine	11. Cocaine	17. Naloxone
3. Barbiturates	12. Imipramine	18. Phenothiazines
4. Chlordiazepoxide	13. LSD	
5. Diazepam	14. Mescaline	
6. Meprobamate	15. Morphine	
7. Nicotine	(and other	
8. Phencyclidine	opiates)	
9. Scopolamine		

Adapted from Overton, 1977.

tion, or it can have a cue function; but can these functions be independent of one another? Table 7-2 suggests that they are.

Consider the relation of discriminability to reinforcing function as a case in point. Drugs that are self-administered can be readily discriminated (alcohol, barbiturates, nicotine, PCP), moderately discriminated (amphetamine, cocaine, the opiates), or poorly discriminated (naloxone). Similarly, drugs that have not been shown to be self-administered and may be aversive, can be readily discriminated (atropine, scopolamine), moderately discriminated (imipramine, mescaline), or poorly discriminated (lithium, phenothiazines). Thus, it appears that cue function does not control the other stimulus functions and vice versa.

Relation to Pharmacologic Class An issue related to such independence among stimulus functions concerns the possibility of a link between discriminability and the pharmacologic properties of different drug groups.

For example, atropine and scopolamine are both anticholinergics and there could be expected to be equally discriminable—and they are, as shown in Table 7-2. Similarly, within the same group are several drugs that have a common pharmacologic property (entries 1, 3, 4, 5, and 6): They all reduce clinical anxiety, as we shall see in Chapter 12. It could be supposed, therefore, that the key to anxiety reduction is somehow related to the fact that these drugs are readily discriminated from saline.

The discriminability of these drugs could be a component in the characteristic clinical activity of these drugs. If this were true, however, all readily discriminated drugs would also be anxiety-reducing. This is clearly not the case; there is no evidence that atropine, nicotine, phen-cyclidine, and scopolamine (entries 2, 7, 8, and 9) are clinically effica-cious in reducing anxiety. Classification as "readily discriminated" would thus generate false positives with regard to the criterion of anx-iety reduction (see Chapter 5). Furthermore, moderately and poorly discriminable drugs fail to cluster into pharmacologically meaningful groupings. Thus, discriminability cannot be directly linked to clinical activity.

STIMULUS CHANGE AND PERFORMANCE CHANGE

The data we have thus far considered leave no doubt that drugs are discriminably different stimuli. This fact has a direct implication for the way in which the behavioral effects of drugs are analyzed.

Virtually all of the procedures in behavioral pharmacology involve first training animals without drug (ND) and then testing them follow-ing drug administration (D). These procedures thus conform to a ND–D paradigm that necessarily incorporates a stimulus change in the ND–D shift.

Now, we know that stimulus change can change ongoing perfor-mance. The ongoing performance of an animal that has been trained to respond in silence, for example, may be disrupted when a noise is introduced; it may, therefore, show a performance decrement. Decre-ment need not necessarily be the rule, however. The phenomenon of rate-dependency suggests that the effects of an added stimulus can de-pend on the baseline rate of the ongoing behavior.

RATE-DEPENDENCY AND STIMULUS CHANGE

McKim (1981) trained animals (in silence) on an FI4 schedule of rein-forcement and, after performance had stabilized, introduced a constant noise of moderate intensity ("white noise"). The use of an FI provided a range of control rates against which the effects of stimulus change could be evaluated (see Chapter 4). A portion of the data obtained are shown in Figure 7–2. There is no question that the introduction of noise changed behavior, and that it did so in a rate-dependent way: low rates were increased; high rates were decreased.

McKim also evaluated the stability of the rate-dependent effect of introducing noise during each of a series of sessions. The results from successive pairs of sessions are shown in Figure 7–3. The introduction of the stimulus obviously produces a rate-dependent effect that is not

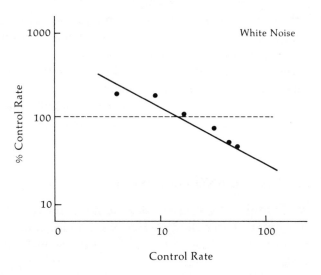

Figure 7–2. Rate-dependent effects due to the introduction of a stimulus change from a no-noise to a noise condition. (Modified from McKim, 1981.)

merely a transient phenomenon. This fact relates directly to the way in which drug effects are viewed.

DRUG EFFECT AND STIMULUS CHANGE

The effects of stimulus change are rate-dependent, and administering a drug produces a stimulus change. It is not surprising, therefore, that a variety of drugs can, and do, produce rate-dependent effects.[4]

Demonstrations of rate-dependency typically involve a ND–D procedure. The complement of this arrangement (D–ND) should, however, also produce stimulus change. A study by Carey (1973) illustrates the point. A control group of rats (given saline before each session) was trained on a DRL schedule of reinforcement. The rats were then given amphetamine before a test session. This is the usual ND–D procedure, and the usual results were obtained: the schedule generated low rates of responding, and amphetamine increased them.

Carey also studied the complementary procedure (D–ND). A second group of rats was also trained on the DRL schedule, but the rats were given amphetamine before each of these training sessions. An injection of saline was then given before a test session. Thus, one group was trained following saline and tested with amphetamine (ND–D), and a second group was trained following amphetamine and tested with saline (D–ND).

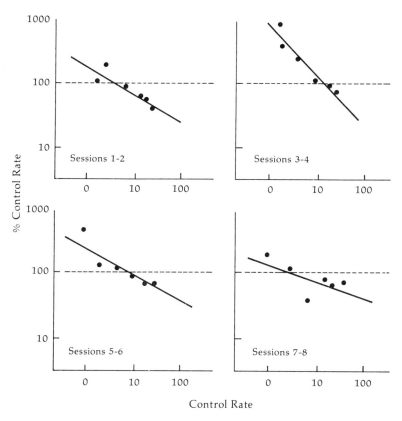

Figure 7–3. Rate-dependent effects of stimulus change in successive pairs of sessions. (Modified from McKim, 1981.)

Carey found that a switch in injections (either saline–amphetamine or amphetamine–saline) produced an increased responding in *both* groups. The response rates are presented in Table 7–3. (The table includes only the data from the first training session, the last session before the switch in treatments, and the test session following this switch.) These data indicate that there was an initial effect of amphetamine in the first training session (8.7 versus 6.3), but that both groups had reached low and equal rates of responding (5.1 Rs/min.) by the last training session. Introduction of amphetamine in the test session reliably increased responding in the first group, (7.9 Rs/min.) as would be expected on the basis of what we know about amphetamine. But the second group also showed an increase in responding (6.2 Rs/min.)

This second result violates common sense but should not be unexpected in light of the foregoing discussion. There is no reason to suppose that amphetamine is not a stimulus and that it can function as any other stimulus can. In this case, a D–ND shift in stimulus conditions increased low response rates just as its complement (ND–D) did.

Note, however, that the complementary shifts did not produce identical effects; the ND–D shift had a greater effect than D–ND. Therefore, amphetamine must be contributing something above and beyond its stimulus effects; if stimulus change were the only factor involved, the effects of the two shifts would have been the same.[5]

These data, in conjunction with those already discussed, indicate that the stimulus effects of drugs can interact with their other effects to determine net outcome. These data also suggest that stimulus effects can interact with dose-dependency.

DOSE DEPENDENCY AND STIMULUS CHANGE

The introduction of drug (ND–D) produces stimulus change; the effect can produce a change in performance. The magnitude of this change in behavior necessarily varies as a function of dose. This is so because of the following effects:

1. The higher the dose, the greater the intensity of the drug as stimulus.
2. The greater the intensity, the greater the ND–D difference.
3. The greater the ND–D difference, the greater the performance change due to stimulus change.

In other words, stimulus change can at least partly control the dose–response functions obtained with ND–D procedures. Furthermore, the nature of these effects on dose–response data may be either incremental or decremental because the effects of stimulus change can be rate-dependent.[6]

Thus, stimulus change turns out to be anything but an incidental effect of drugs. Indeed, it can be a powerful factor in the determination

Table 7–3

Session	Condition*		Rs/min	
	Group 1	Group 2	Group 1	Group 2
First Training	S	A	6.3	8.7
Last Training	S	A	5.1	5.1
Test	A	S	7.9	6.2

*S-saline; A-amphetamine.
From Carey, 1973.

of any drug effect. We are therefore obligated to examine explicitly its contribution to the various phenomena we shall be considering in the chapters that lie ahead. For the moment, however, let us consider some more immediate implications of the cue functions of drugs.

IMPLICATIONS OF CUE FUNCTIONS

THE STUDY OF MEMORY

We have seen that a shift in drug condition can produce stimulus change and that, under some conditions, this change can produce a performance decrement. Decrements of this kind can, however, be interpreted in another way. They can be, and have been, assumed to be a reflection of a disruption of memory processes. That is, a decrement in the ND–D paradigm could reflect a drug-induced disruption of a retrieval process necessary for recall; a decrement in the D–ND paradigm could reflect a drug-induced disruption of an initial encoding process that is also necessary for subsequent recall. It is a common report that excessive alcohol consumption, for example, leads to subsequent failure to remember what took place during intoxication (D–ND); conversely, intoxication often interferes with the ability to recall memories that would certainly be available prior to alcohol consumption (ND–D).

The problem with interpreting these deficits as those involving memory processes is that they are not definitive. The deficits could be due to either stimulus change *or* to a drug-induced disruption of memory processes. How, then, can we distinguish between these two equally plausible alternatives? The trick is to eliminate the possibility of stimulus change, by studying the effects of a D–D arrangement. If memory impairment occurs under these circumstances, it cannot be due to to stimulus change because none is involved. Table 7–4 explains why this is so.

Table 7–4

Group	Train	Test	Possible interference with memory?*	Possible stimulus change?
A	D	ND	Yes; in training	Yes
B	ND	D	Yes; in test	Yes
C	D	D	Yes; in either training *or* test	No

*Interference would be indicated by a deficit relative to performance of a ND–ND control group in test.

Suppose animals are trained while they are drugged and then are tested without drug (Group A). If they were inferior to a ND–ND group in this test, we might say that the drug had interfered with the original encoding of memory. But this result could just as well be due to stimulus change. Similarly, if animals are trained without drug but are tested following drug (Group B), we might conclude that the drug interfered with recall from memory. But this effect, too, could just as well be due to stimulus change.

Now consider Group C. A deficit obtained in these animals could be due to either an interference with encoding or recall but not to stimulus change, because stimulus change cannot have occurred. Furthermore, the data from Groups A and B can be used for further analysis of our results. This analysis is schematized in Table 7–5.

If a deficit is obtained in Group C, we can conclude that the drug has somehow interfered with memory processes because the results cannot be due to stimulus change. Given this, if a comparable deficit is also obtained in Group B (but not Group A), we can conclude that the deficit seen in Group C is due to a drug-induced interference with recall. Conversely, a deficit in Group A (but not Group B) would indicate that the drug interfered with the original encoding of memory. Finally, with the result shown at the bottom of the table, we might conclude that the drug interfered with both recall and encoding processes.[7, 8]

Drug-induced deficits are often attributed to disrupted memory processes in the absence of the necessary D–D procedure. Indeed, the drugs most often cited as producing memory disturbances are also those that are most readily discriminated from saline (entries 1, 2, 3, 4, 5, 6, and 9 in Table 7–2). These are the same drugs, however, that would be ex-

Table 7–5

Group	Deficit relative to ND–ND in test?	Interpretation: Interference is with
C (D–D)	Yes	Encoding or recall
B (ND–D)	Yes	Recall but not encoding
A (D–ND)	No	
B (ND–D)	No	Encoding but not recall
A (D–ND)	Yes	
B (ND–D)	Yes	Both encoding and recall
A (D–ND)	Yes	

pected to produce the greatest performance decrements because the D–ND (or ND–D) difference is greatest. Conclusions about memory deficits caused by these drugs should, in the absence of the crucial D–D comparison, be viewed with skepticism.

HABITUATION AND TOLERANCE

To conclude our study of the cue functions of drugs, let us take a preliminary look at a phenomenon called *habituation*.

The initial presentation of a stimulus has an effect on the organism that may be reflected in a change in some physiologic process (e.g., heart rate), the elicitation of an orienting reaction (e.g., "looking" at the stimulus), a modification of ongoing behavior, or any one of a variety of other indices. Repeated presentation of the same stimulus leads to a gradual diminution in the magnitude of the initial response. This waning, due solely to stimulus presentation, is called habituation.

Habituation has a formal similarity to another phenomenon, *tolerance*. In this case, initial administration of a drug produces some effect, but it too may decrease with repeated drug administration. This waning of drug effect is called tolerance.

Habituation and tolerance have traditionally been viewed as distinctly different processes. However, because drugs do have demonstrable stimulus properties, the suspicion arises that these two analogous phenomena may be linked in some way. Might the waning of drug effect (tolerance) in fact represent an instance of the waning of a stimulus effect (habituation)? Might the processes actually be the same?

We cannot answer these questions until we have considered the phenomenon of tolerance itself. This is the topic of Section III.

NOTES

1. A more detailed discussion of many of the ideas discussed here can be found in an elegant article by Schuster and Balster (1977).
2. A much more thorough discussion of these procedures and their implications can be found in an article by Overton (1974).
3. The completeness of the discrimination has led to the idea that the animals are "dissociated" from their normal "state" while drugged. In fact, phenomena of these kinds are often called "state-dependent." Be that as it may, the question of whether these "state-dependencies" are due to processes that are fundamentally different from those involved in ordinary discriminations is an open one.

4. The role of stimulus change in producing rate-dependency suggests that, under matched conditions, readily discriminable drugs (greater stimulus change) might be characterized by greater rate-dependency than drugs that are poorly discriminated (smaller stimulus change). This prospect has not yet been examined experimentally.

5. Other drugs have been shown to produce asymmetrical effects in that the consequence of an ND–D shift is not equal to the effect of D–ND; see Berger and Stein (1969).

6. Any drug has the potential of producing stimulus change and, as a result, rate-dependent effects. This fact implies that rate-dependency is due, at least in part, to the nonspecific stimulus properties of different drugs; see McKim (1981).

7. An excellent example of the way in which such procedures can be used to study memory processes can be found in an article by Patel, Ciofalo, and Iorio (1979).

8. This analysis presupposes that deficits in test are not due to a simple debilitation of the animal by drug. For example, if the measure of recall were suppression due to punishment, a deficit would then be reflected in an increase in responding (less suppression) and could not be attributed to debilitation.

Section 3
The Phenomenon of Tolerance

REPEATED ADMINISTRATION OF a drug can lead to a loss of its initial effect. In persons who rarely drink, for example, the first martini typically packs a substantial wallop. Seasoned drinkers are, however, much less affected; they find that it takes more than one martini to equal the effect of the first drink. This diminution of effect is called *tolerance.*

The phenomenon of tolerance is characterized by three features: It occurs in response to repeated drug administration; it is revealed in a loss of effect relative to initial impact; and it results in greater amounts of drug being required to reinstate that initial effect.

The complement of tolerance is called *sensitization.* Sensitization is an increase in drug effect relative to initial impact. It too is a consequence of repeated drug administration but differs from tolerance in that less, not more, drug is required to reinstate the initial effect.

However, the behavioral analysis of tolerance and sensitization amounts to more than a demonstration of altered drug effect due to repeated administration; we shall consider the reasons why this is so in Chapter 8. Furthermore, these changes do not inhere solely in the pharmacologic properties of drugs. Indeed, environmental factors can be major determinants of outcome, as we shall see in Chapter 9.

Chapter 8

Basic Factors in Tolerance

THERE ARE TWO basic ways in which tolerance can be determined. One procedure tests three groups of animals; a schematic is given in Table 8–1.[1] For this procedure the first group, SS, is given a series of control injections, typically saline (S). The number of injections may range from as few as 1 or as many as n. This group is given the same final injection prior to a test for behavioral effect.

Group SD follows this same sequence except that drug (D) is given prior to test. On the other hand, Group DD is given drug throughout the sequence. Thus, Group SS provides a control for the effects of repeated treatment without drug, whereas Group SD provides an index of the effect of drug given for the first time. The effect of drug following the final injection given Group DD indicates whether tolerance has occurred. If tolerance has occurred, the test data for Group DD should approach that of Group SS and differ from that of Group SD. Complete

Table 8–1

Group	Prior injections 1 2 3. . .n	Final injection
SS (control)	S S S S	S
SD	S S S S	D
DD	D D D D	D

tolerance would amount to the equivalent of "no drug" condition; that is, the effect seen in Group DD would not differ from that for Group SS.[2]

A second procedure involves a single group of animals rather than three. In this case, the effects of saline and of drug are first determined in separate tests. A series of drug injections are then given, and the first test is repeated. This procedure thus conforms to the outline in Table 8–2.

TEMPORAL PARAMETERS

Tolerance can have a very definite time course. Let us consider the effects of two drugs, nicotine and morphine, in order to illustrate the different temporal characteristics that tolerance to different drugs may have.

EFFECTS OF NICOTINE

The experiment we shall consider involved a measure of motor activity (Stolerman, Fink, and Jarvik, 1973). The procedure used corresponds to the general format shown in Table 8–1; in this case only one prior injection was given (i.e., $n = 1$). Thus, Group DD received only two injections. In addition, there were several subgroups within Group DD. One of these was given the second injection one-half hour after the first injection, the second one an hour later, and so on. The effects of nicotine on the motor activity of these subgroups and of Groups SS and SD are shown in Figure 8–1.

Nicotine given for the first time (Group SD) clearly decreased activity relative to control levels (Group SS). The overall level of tolerance due to a prior injection of nicotine (Group DD) is thus reflected as a shift in activity away from Group SD and toward Group SS. (Note the label on the ordinate.) More significant, however, is the temporal dependency in this shift.

An injection of nicotine given one-half hour before the test injection produces little tolerance. That is, the subgroup from Group DD at the

Table 8–2

First tests	Interpolated injections 1 2 3. . .n	Final tests
S and D in separate tests	D D D D	S and D in separate tests

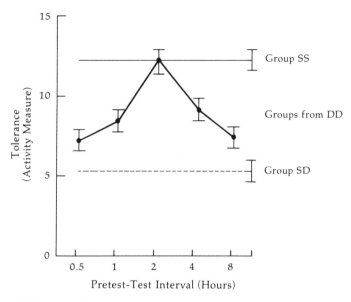

Figure 8–1. Temporal characteristics of tolerance to nicotine; see text for details. (From Stolerman, Fink, and Jarvik, 1973.)

lower left of the figure differs little from Group SD. On the other hand, the degree of tolerance increases and then declines as the interval between injections is increased.

There are two important lessons to be learned from these data. First, we might intuitively expect level of tolerance to be maximal at the shortest interval because this is when most drug is present. That naive expectation is not confirmed, however. This behavioral index of tolerance must therefore be dependent on processes other than those directly related to levels of drug.

Second, a failure to evaluate a range of intervals could have led us to the conclusion that little, if any, tolerance occurs at all. If the tests had been too early (at a pretest–test interval less than one-half hour) or too late (at an interval greater than eight hours), the fact of tolerance might have been overlooked completely. As a general rule, then, the examination of temporal parameters can be crucial.

EFFECTS OF MORPHINE

The time course of tolerance in Figure 8–1 is brief. That this is not necessarily so was dramatically illustrated in a study by Kornetsky and Bain (1968).

In this experiment, laboratory rats could terminate an electric shock by emitting a prescribed response. The intensity of the shock was gradually increased until the animals responded. Thus, responding indicated a threshold for escape behavior.

Morphine is a potent analgesic; it therefore increased the threshold. That is, higher shock intensities were required to engender the escape response. A second injection of morphine produced essentially the same effect a day later; there was no tolerance with a one-day pretest–test interval. However, when different animals were tested at longer intervals, tolerance was found from one to four *months* later.

These findings parallel those shown in Figure 8–1 in that tolerance is initially minimal and increases at longer intervals. But the time scale for this parallel is enormously different: tolerance to the effects of nicotine on motor activity is measured in hours, whereas that to the effects of morphine on shock escape is measured in months.

This difference brings us to an important issue. Obviously, incorrect conclusions could be drawn about different drugs by an inappropriate choice of test interval. The conclusion that tolerance characterizes one drug, but not another, thus requires extensive exploration of temporal parameters.

BIPHASIC DOSE–RESPONSE FUNCTIONS

The need for extensive evaluation applies as well to another parameter, one that we have repeatedly encountered earlier: the dose of drug studied.

We know that an initially increasing dose–response function will inevitably invert and decrease at high dose levels. This fact can lead to very misguided conclusions about tolerance. Figure 8–2 indicates why this can be so.

Suppose a range of doses are evaluated in an initial behavioral test, with the resulting function at the left of the figure. Now suppose that these same animals are given a series of injections of drug at some dose and that the dose–response function is then redetermined in a second test.

If tolerance has occurred as a consequence of the injections given between tests, then the function will have been shifted in the direction of higher doses. That shift defines tolerance.

Now suppose that, instead, only one dose of drug had been studied. If dose *B* had been chosen, we would conclude, correctly, that tolerance had taken place. The effect of drug in the second test is less than that

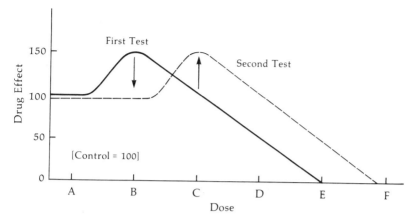

Figure 8–2. Schematic dose–response functions prior to (left-hand curve) and after (right-hand curve) interpolated injections.

obtained in the first, as indicated by the arrow. On the other hand, we would have reached just the opposite conclusion if dose *C* had been chosen. In this case, the effect of drug is greater in the second test, as indicated by the second arrow. In short, actual tolerance can produce an *apparent* sensitization in the absence of dose–response data. A concrete example is given in Figure 8–3.

These data were obtained from a study of the effects of morphine on rates of responding maintained by a nondiscriminated avoidance schedule (Holtzman, 1974). The dose-dependency obtained in the first test is biphasic, as indicated by the solid curve. That is, relative to the control value given at the lower left of the the panel, morphine had an incremental and then a decremental effect on responding.

The dose–response function obtained following a series of interpolated injections is indicated by the dashed curve. Tolerance has occurred, as shown by the shift in the dose–response curve in the direction of higher doses. Furthermore, this conclusion could have been drawn on the basis of a study of any one of the doses less than 10.0 mg/kg. But if only that high dose had been chosen, apparent sensitization would have been the result.

When the basic dose–response function is biphasic, tolerance can only be inferred from dose–response data because, in their absence, true tolerance can easily be confused with apparent sensitization. The same rule applies to true sensitization, as can be seen by again referring to Figure 8–3.

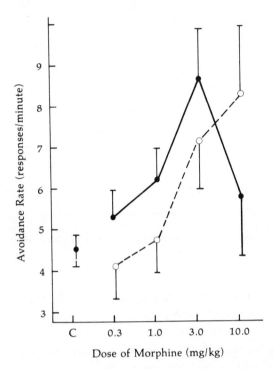

Figure 8–3. Dose–response functions for the effects of morphine on nondiscriminated avoidance. The solid curve is the function obtained prior to interpolated injections; the dashed curve is the function obtained after them. (From Holtzman, 1974.)

Imagine that the effects of the initial injections are characterized by the dashed curve. The effect of interpolated injections (the solid curve) will thus be a shift to lower doses. This is a reflection of true sensitization. But if only the 10.0 mg/kg dose were studied, the true sensitization will generate an apparent tolerance (i.e., there will be less of an effect of this dose following interpolated injections). As we have seen so often before, single-dose data can lead to major error.

MONOPHASIC DOSE–RESPONSE FUNCTIONS

As we noted in Chapter 3, virtually all of the drugs we shall be considering generate biphasic dose–response functions of behavioral effect. However, the material we have just considered is also pertinent to monophasic functions.

Before initiation of a series of interpolated injections in studying tolerance, a dose–response function must first be obtained to determine whether the drug under study is truly monophasic in its activity. Then, following interpolated doses, a rightward shift in the function will indicate tolerance.

Recall that monophasic dose–response functions of behavioral effect are always decremental; one of these is indicated by the solid line in Figure 8–4. (Note the use of logarithmic dose units to obtain linear functions; see Figure 3–4.) The dashed line labeled *II* is a hypothetical function obtained following interpolated doses. Tolerance is evident in the shift to higher doses. Furthermore, all doses that initially produce a decrement are less effective following the development of tolerance. Thus, apparent sensitization cannot occur. (The ED_{50} will be discussed later.)

True sensitization can, however, be the result of interpolated doses, as indicated by the dashed function labeled *I*. In this case, all doses now produce a greater decremental effect, so that a tolerance that is only apparent cannot occur.

This illustration assumes that the form of the dose–response functions following interpolated doses is unchanged. There is no guarantee, however, that an initially monophasic function might not become biphasic despite an overall rightward shift. Under these circumstances, apparent sensitization could occur as a consequence of tolerance and

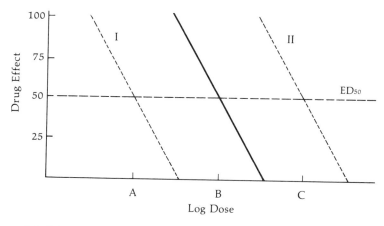

Figure 8–4. Schematic dose–response functions indicating the effect of drug prior to interpolated injections (the solid line) as well as after them (the dashed lines). The line labeled *I* indicates that sensitization has occurred; the one labeled *II* indicates tolerance. The ED_{50} is indicated by the horizontal dashed line.

vice versa. As a general rule, then, dose–response functions should be determined both before and after interpolated doses.

MED AND ED_{50}

As noted in Chapter 3, one way of characterizing dose–response information is to rely on a single index such as the MED or ED_{50}. The shift in dose–response function due to tolerance or sensitization can also be characterized in this way. Let us again consider Figure 8–4 to illustrate how this can be done. The middle dose–response function is based on an initial determination and indicates that the ED_{50} is equal to dose B; that is, dose B is the value at which the horizontal dashed line (ED_{50}) intersects the dose–response function. Tolerance (line II) results in an increase in the ED_{50} to dose C, whereas sensitization results in a decrease to dose A. These same relationships would hold, of course, for the MED (or any other single value used to describe drug effect) so long as the functions are parallel.

The effect of a change in the form of the pre- and post-tolerance functions is shown in Figure 8–5. (In this case, the parallelism has broken down. Other changes in form could result in distortions comparable to the one under discussion.) The MED obtained pre-tolerance is dose A, and the post-tolerance MED is also dose A; the pre-tolerance ED_{50} is dose B, and the post-tolerance ED_{50} is dose C. Accordingly, if the MED is used as our index of tolerance, we will falsely conclude that tolerance has not taken place (no change in MEDs). If, on the other hand, the ED_{50} is used, we will correctly conclude that tolerance has indeed occurred (the shift in ED_{50} from B to C). We cannot know all this, of course, without the dose–response data. Actual dose–response information is therefore far more useful than are derived indices. Furthermore, the situation described in Figure 8–5 is not a fanciful one, as we shall see in the following chapter.[3]

NOTES

1. Much of the material discussed here and in the following chapter is derived from an outstanding review by Corfield-Sumner and Stolerman (1978).
2. As a general rule, increasing the number of prior injections (n) can be expected to increase the level of tolerance. This means that a lack of tolerance could be due not to an intrinsic property of the drug

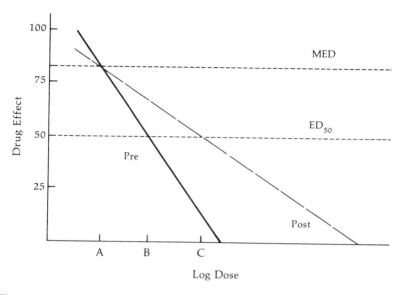

Figure 8–5. Schematic dose–response functions indicating the effect of a lack of parallel-ism in the function obtained before interpolated injections *(pre)* and after them *(post)*.

being studied but to an insufficient *n*. The conclusion that a drug does not produce tolerance can, therefore, be an artifact of a faulty proce-dure just as negative conclusions about the lack of other effects can be due to a failure to study an adequate dose range.

3. **Cross-tolerance** refers to the substitution of one drug for another without a loss of tolerance. Tolerance developed to drug *A* might not be lost if drug *B* were substituted for it, but would be lost if drug *C* were substituted. Thus, cross-tolerance provides a way in which drugs can be grouped in terms of a shared property. A drug that will substitute for an opiate, for example, is likely to be addicting in its own right.

Chapter 9

Environmental Factors in Tolerance

ONE OF THE sets of data discussed in Chapter 7 was that reported by Carey; his study involved a group of animals exposed to a DRL schedule in a series of sessions before each of which amphetamine was given. In another aspect of this experiment, the motor activity of the same animals was also measured. In these tests, Carey determined levels of locomotor activity following amphetamine (in one group of animals) or saline (in another).

The values in Table 9–1 are those obtained in the first and last sessions of the four-week series.

As noted in Chapter 7, the effect of amphetamine in the first session was, as expected, an increase in DRL responding. The difference, shown in parentheses, was 2.4 responses per minute. On the other hand, the difference in responding was zero by the last session. Given the infor-

Table 9–1

Measure	Injection	First session	Last session
DRL	Saline	6.3 (2.4)	5.1 (0)
(Responses/min)	Amphetamine	8.7	5.1
Activity	Saline	27.6 (36.6)	22.5 (39.1)
(Counts/min)	Amphetamine	64.2	61.6

From Carey, 1973.

mation in the previous chapter, we might conclude that this is an instance of tolerance to the effects of amphetamine. Such a result is not surprising because animals do become tolerant to amphetamine. What *is* surprising about the data in Table 9–1 are the data for motor activity. In the first session there is an increase due to amphetamine (equal to 36.6 counts per minute), but by the last session, tolerance has not occurred: The difference is as robust as it was initially (39.1 counts per minute). In short, evidence for the expected tolerance appears in one measure (DRL) but not in the second (activity).

It is important to bear in mind that the data both for DRL and for activity were taken from the same animals given either saline (one group) or a constant dose of amphetamine (the second group) over the course of a series of sessions. Thus, the animals are tolerant to the effects of drug when one measure is used but are apparently not tolerant when another measure is used. The nature of this differential effect is the subject of this chapter.

TOLERANCE AND REINFORCEMENT DENSITY

There is a major difference in the behaviors involved in Carey's experiment: one behavior (DRL) is maintained by reinforcement, whereas the second (activity) is not. The initial effect of amphetamine is to increase behavior in both cases, but only in the case of DRL is there a specific consequence of this change. In particular, the increase in responding necessarily leads to a reduction in the rate at which reinforcements occur because the DRL schedule specifies low response rates as a condition of reinforcement. Thus, there is a reduction in reinforcement density in the case of DRL and, necessarily, no such reduction in the case of activity.

REINFORCEMENT LOSS

The effect of amphetamine on DRL performance involves a reduction in reinforcement density. That is, the environmental contingency (the DRL reinforcement schedule) controls behavior (low response rate), but the drug (amphetamine) changes the behavior (increases rates) so that responding is less frequently reinforced. If we know anything at all about the behavior of organisms, we know that their behaviors are adjusted to reinforcement contingencies. It is therefore not surprising that response rates decline just as they would if reinforcement contingency were changed, not by drug effect but by some other means. In other words, the tolerance evident in Table 9–1 may reflect an adjustment to the effects of amphetamine that corrects for the loss of reinforcement.

This idea was first advanced by Schuster and Zimmerman (1961) in a report of data essentially identical to those summarized in Table 9–1. Schuster, Dockens, and Woods (1966) later amplified the point by comparing the effects of repeated injections of amphetamine on behaviors maintained by different schedules of reinforcement, with the following findings:

1. When amphetamine initially increased response rates *and* reduced reinforcement density, tolerance occurred.
2. When amphetamine initially increased response rates but did *not* reduce reinforcement density, tolerance did *not* occur.

These findings suggest that an initial effect will wane (tolerate) in the face of repeated drug administration only if there is a reduction in reinforcement density. The occurrence of tolerance does not appear to be dependent on either schedule as such or on an initial increase in response rate that does not also engender a reduction in reinforcement. This latter result parallels that seen in motor activity: there is an increase in responding; there is no consequence of this increase (there is no reinforcement to be lost) and thus no sign of tolerance.

INJECTION–TEST INTERACTIONS: THE B-A PROCEDURE

There is another procedure for examining the general idea that tolerance to the effect of a drug is contingent upon the loss in reinforcements that the drug produces. This procedure is a particularly useful one because it involves not different kinds of behavior (e.g., activity versus DRL) but the same behavior studied in relation to the time of drug injection.

The basic comparison involves injecting animals with drug either before or after the test sessions. Over the course of several sessions, animals given drug before the sessions—the B animals—will have had a series of exposures to drug *during* the test; animals given drug after each session—the A animals—will have had the *same* exposure to drug but never during test.

If tolerance is solely a consequence of drug action, then both B and A animals should show comparable tolerance. However, if environmental factors interact with pharmacologic factors in determining tolerance, the B and A groups should differ. More particularly, if reduction in reinforcement density is a significant element in determining tolerance, then the B animals should show greater tolerance than A animals because only the B animals will have been exposed to reinforcement loss while drugged. On the other hand, if this drug–environment interaction is not critical, both groups should show comparable tolerance because both will have received identical injections. Only the relation of injection to test will differ, and if that interaction is not relevant, levels of tolerance should be the same.

The B-A procedure was introduced by Chen (1968) in a study of the effects of alcohol on performance in a maze. Rats were first trained to perform reliably in the maze, and then a series of alcohol injections was begun. One group (B) received injections before each test session in the maze, whereas the second (A) received injections after each session.

Chen found that the initial effect of alcohol in the B animals was a marked deterioration of performance and a consequent loss of reinforcements; the animals earned about 30 reinforcements under control conditions and about 1 reinforcement following the first injection of alcohol. By the fourth session, each preceded by injection, these B animals showed clear tolerance to the initially depressant effects of alcohol; they earned 26 reinforcements (87% of the control value of 30 reinforcements).

All that this result means is that tolerance to alcohol can develop; the crucial question is whether animals given alcohol *after* each session (the A animals) were or were not tolerant. This question was answered by giving these animals alcohol not *after* the session but *before* it for the first time. Chen found that the performance of these A animals was seriously depressed; they earned only 3 reinforcements (10% of the control value). Bear in mind that, at the time of test, both B and A animals had had identical injections—that the only difference between them was the relation of injection to test—yet only the B animals showed tolerance. These relationships are summarized in Table 9–2.

The general nature of these results with alcohol have been extended to the effects of amphetamine on DRL responding (Campbell and Sei-

Table 9–2

Group	Alcohol injections	Reinforcements in session 4 (percentage of control value)
B	Before sessions 1–4	87%
A	After sessions 1–3; *before* session 4	10%

den, 1973). As would be expected on the basis of the findings already discussed, this study indicated that drug action at the time of testing (and reinforcement loss due to the increase in response rate produced by amphetamine) produced tolerance, whereas there was little if any in the A animals.

The study by Campbell and Seiden involved increased responding due to amphetamine. Comparable results have been obtained in a situation in which this same drug produced a *decrease* in responding.

Amphetamine is anorexigenic; that is, it decreases food intake. When tolerance to this decrease in responding (eating) was evaluated with the B-A procedure (Carlton and Wolgin, 1971), it was again found that drug action at the time of testing (i.e., the opportunity to eat) led to tolerance, whereas the same dose of amphetamine given after each test did not.[2] This finding adds generality to the previous findings in that both increased (DRL) and decreased responding (eating), both induced by the same drug, show differential tolerance with the B-A technique. In both instances, exposure to drug at the time of test profoundly augmented the degree of tolerance. We shall explore this general conclusion further in the following section.

ENVIRONMENTAL SPECIFICITY

Results of several experiments by Siegel (1978a, 1978b) extend our conclusion that degree of tolerance to the same drug can differ under different circumstances. The data already discussed implicate an environmental contingency (reinforcement loss during drug action); Siegel's experiments do not involve reinforcement contingencies as such, yet his results point in the same direction.

These studies involved injections given in two distinctly different environments. One of these was the room in which the animals were tested; the second, "non-test" environment was the room in which the animals were housed. The two rooms differed with respect to both ambient noise and level of illumination.

One group of animals (I) was given a series of injections of morphine in the test environment; on different days these same animals received saline in the non-test environment. A second group (II) underwent the opposite regimen; they received saline in the test environment and, on different days, morphine in the non-test environment.

The effect of morphine that Siegel recorded was the increase in body temperature that this drug can produce. The first injection was given to the Group I animals in the test environment in which body temperature was recorded. It produced an increase of a little over 1.0°C above normal body temperature. This value (1.1°) is entered in parentheses for Group I in Test 1 (Table 9–3). The M entered next to this value indicates that these animals had received morphine; the lower entry, S, indicates that they also received saline on another day in the non-test environment. The series of subsequent tests (2 through 5) reveal a gradual waning of the initial hyperthermic effect of morphine (to an elevation of only 0.1° in Test 5).

The Group II animals received the same sequence of injections as had Group I, the only difference being that morphine was administered in the non-test environment (and saline in the test environment) during the period occupied by the initial four tests. These treatments are indicated by the M and S entries in the third and fourth rows of Table 9–3.

If the development of tolerance were solely dependent on morphine, the animals in Group II would be expected to show a small increase in temperature comparable to the 0.1° rise shown by Group I in Test 5. But this result was not obtained. Despite the identical prior series of drug treatments, these animals showed a rise of 0.9°, a value that is nearly equal to that due to the initial injection (1.1° for Group I under Test 1).

This result means that the effects of injections given in one environment (the non-test environment for Group II) do not completely transfer to another environment (the test environment). In other words, tolerance developed in an environment that is the *same* as that in which it was tested (Group I) is greater than that developed when the two environments are *different* (Group II). The data shown in Figure 9–1 illustrate the same point: the "same" animals are more tolerant to the hyperthermic effects of morphine despite the fact that both groups had received identical injections of drug prior to test (Siegel, 1978b). Recall

Table 9–3

Group	Environment	Test 1	2	3	4	5
I	Test	M(1.1)	M(0.7)	M(0.5)	M(0.4)	M(0.1)
	Non-test	S	S	S	S	S
II	Test	S	S	S	S	M(0.9)*
	Non-test	M	M	M	M	S

*First injection of morphine in test environment.
Values estimated from Siegel, 1978a.

that tolerance is shown by a *reduction* in the temperature rise due to morphine (i.e., by less hyperthermia).

Siegel has extended the analysis to include tolerance to the analgesia initially produced by morphine. These results lead to the same conclusion: The environment in which injections occur can largely determine level of tolerance.

Does the fact that tolerance can be environmentally specific mean that, as a general rule, tolerance is entirely dependent on environmental control? This question brings us to the distinction between physiologic and behavioral tolerance.

BEHAVIORAL AND PHYSIOLOGIC TOLERANCE

The traditional interpretation of tolerance is that a drug initially induces some metabolic process that subsequently reduces the drug's own activity. Barbiturates, for example, are known to activate enzymes involved in the metabolism of the barbiturates themselves; a second injection of barbiturates, therefore, has less effect because of accelerated metabolism and excretion of the drug.

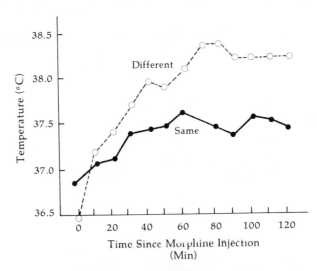

Figure 9-1. Time course of hyperthermia due to morphine in two groups of animals that had received a series of identical prior injections. One group (the "same" animals) had received these injections in an environment that was the same as the one in which they were tested and the data in the figure recorded. The second group (the "different" animals) had received prior injections in an environment different from the one in which they were tested. The "same" animals are clearly more tolerant. (From Siegel, 1978b.)

The enzyme induction produced by barbiturates is an example of what is called *physiologic tolerance*. That is, the phenomenon of tolerance is due to some endogenous process that is independent of environmental circumstance. Such an account is obviously incomplete, as the data just discussed make clear.

These latter data are usually included under the subject of *behavioral tolerance* because they involve variables that control behavior (environmental stimuli, schedule of reinforcement, loss of reinforcement). However, the fact that behavioral factors are potent ones does not mean that physiologic tolerance does not occur. (After all, tolerance does occur in isolated tissues to which behavioral variables can hardly be relevant.) Rather, it is more sensible to suppose that these two sets of factors—physiologic and behavioral—interact to determine net outcome: the phenomenon of tolerance itself. Because, as we have repeatedly seen, experimental detail dictates experimental outcome, it is certain that behavioral variables will predominate in some circumstances and that physiologic variables will predominate in others. The question is not whether one set of variables operates to the exclusion of the other but how these two act in concert. As it happens, we can best amplify the point by considering a study that does not involve tolerance at all.

Clody and Beer (1975) were interested in how long the effects of a single dose of a drug lasted. This drug was known to specifically reduce discriminated avoidance responding (see Chapter 13). They gave the drug to a group of animals and then tested the animals at each of several times following injection. That is, the same animals were tested one day after injection, then tested again seven days after injection, then again fourteen days after injection, and so on. The results are shown in Table 9–4. The values entered in the table are percentages of pre-drug levels of avoidance for the same animals given repeated tests. Thus, one day after injection, performance deteriorated from 100% to 49% and had not completely recovered four weeks later (66%).

This experiment studied a physiologic process—clearance of a single dose over time. The data in Table 9–4 indicate that the drug had not

Table 9–4

Days following injection				
1	7	14	21	28
49	60	56	55	66

Adapted from Clody and Beer, 1975.

been completely eliminated at four weeks after a single injection—or do they?

Clody and Beer also studied separate groups that were injected and then given a single test at different times following injection (one group was injected and tested the next day, a second group was injected and tested one week later, and so on). The results of this experiment are shown in Table 9–5. In this instance, performance deteriorated to a level identical to that seen in the first experiment (49% of control), but unlike that in the first experiment, recovery was found to be essentially complete in three to four weeks. How long is the drug active?

The data reflect not only a physiologic process but a behavioral one as well. Clearly, repeated testing (Table 9–4) introduced behavioral processes that substantially prolonged the apparent duration of a physiologic process: excretion of drug. The question of how long the drug is active can be answered only in terms that specify the conditions of the experiment and thereby the extent to which physiologic and behavioral processes may interact to generate overall outcome. Simple questions about duration of action—like simple questions about tolerance—are not meaningful in the absence of a delineation of the relative contributions of the processes involved.

SENSITIZATION

As noted in Chapter 8, sensitization is the complement of tolerance. If there is behavioral tolerance, is there also behavioral sensitization?

Unfortunately, there are few data pertinent to the question. One study does, however, suggest that behavioral sensitization can be obtained. In this experiment (Kuribara, 1980), rats were given amphetamine before each of ten sessions in which nondiscriminated avoidance responding was measured (Group 1). A second group (Group 2) was given the same dose of amphetamine *after* each of the initial nine sessions and then, for the first time, was injected *before* the tenth session. The experiment thus follows the B-A procedure: Group 1 corresponds to the B treatment and Group 2 to the A.

Table 9–5

Days following injection				
1	7	14	21	28
49	50	66	89	91

Adapted from Clody and Beer, 1975.

The results of the study are shown in Figure 9–2. The data in panel *A* indicate that amphetamine given for the first time to Group 1 produced an increase in responding that was sustained throughout the two hours of the session. Drug was given before this session and before each of the subsequent nine. The effect of the same dose of amphetamine in the last session is shown in panel *B*. Apparently, a sensitization due to the intervening pre-session injections has developed.

But what about the effects of giving amphetamine after each session preceding the last? The answer is provided in panel *C*. In this case, amphetamine was given before the session for the first time; the animals had received injections *after* each of the preceding nine sessions.

The data in panel *C* suggest that sensitization has occurred in that response levels are greater than those in panel *A*. Furthermore, it appears that there was an environmental interaction in that levels of responding are greater in panel *B* than in panel *C;* that is, nine injections given before each session had a greater effect than nine injections given after each session. It therefore seems that sensitization, like tolerance, is greater when injections are combined with behavioral measurement.

Let us pause at this point to raise two important questions: Has behavioral sensitization truly been demonstrated? Alternatively, might the data in Figure 9–2 represent a shift in the dose–response curve due to tolerance, not sensitization?

The material discussed in the previous chapter (see Figures 8–2 and 8–3) certainly indicate that the answer to our second question could be affirmative. However, whether sensitization has truly been demonstrated cannot be determined in the absence of dose-response data.

DOSE–RESPONSE FUNCTION AND THE B-A PROCEDURE

The necessity for dose–response data in determining sensitization reflects another aspect of the always-critical matter of dose determination. We shall consider the dose–response function as it applies specifically to the B-A procedure.

The experiment that we shall now consider is one reported by Tang and Falk (1978). In this study, deprived rats were trained to lever press for food on a FI1 schedule of reinforcement. They were then given various doses of phenobarbital, and a dose–response function was determined. Phenobarbital reduced response rates and thereby engendered a loss of reinforcement. The dose-dependent character of this loss in reinforcements is shown at the left of Figure 9–3. For example, the dose

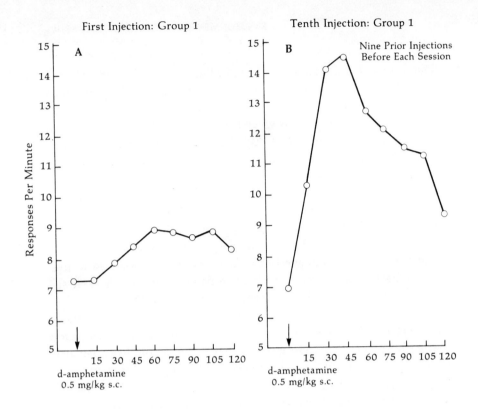

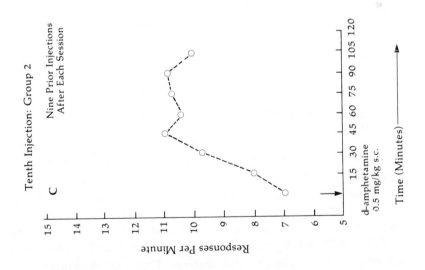

Figure 9–2. Time course of effects of amphetamine on nondiscriminated avoidance responding. The initial incremental effect of 0.5 mg/kg is shown in panel *A* (Group 1). The effect of nine prior injections given *before* each session is shown in panel *B;* apparent sensitization is the result (Group 1). The apparent sensitization due to nine injections given *after* each of the preceding sessions is shown in panel *C* (Group 2); it is less than that shown in panel *B*. (Modified from Kuribara, 1980.)

of 80.0 mg/kg reduced responding and eventuated in a decrease in the number of reinforcements from about 170 following saline (zero on the abscissa) to about 100.

Following this initial dose–response determination, all animals were given a series of injections at a dose level of 80.0 mg/kg (the interpolated dose level indicated at the top of Figure 9–3). One-half of the animals received these injections before each daily session—the B group; the second half received them after each session—the A group. Thus, the drug was active during the sessions for the B animals but not during those for the A animals.

Dose–response functions for the two groups were again determined after 13 injections of 80.0 mg/kg had been given; these functions are shown at the right of Figure 9–3 (the dashed curve *A* describes the data for the A animals; the solid curve *B* is for the B animals).

On the basis of the data discussed earlier in this chapter, we would expect that the B animals would show tolerance, whereas the A animals would show little if any. Most of the data we have already considered

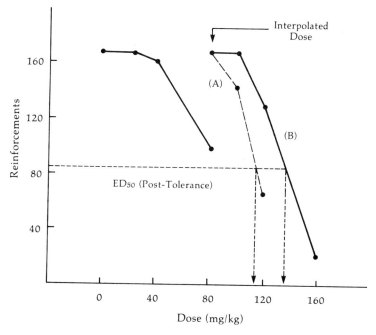

Figure 9–3. Dose–response functions before (at the left) and after (at the right) tolerance due to injections given after each of the interpolated sessions *(A)* or before each of them *(B)*. (Redrawn from Tang and Falk, 1978.)

are, however, based on a single-dose level given (1) to produce an initial effect, (2) throughout an interpolated tolerance period and (3) again during test. The 80.0-mg/kg dose corresponds to this regimen, but as Figure 9-3 shows, there was no difference in tolerance in the A and B groups. That is, both groups showed complete tolerance to the initial effect of 80.0 mg/kg of drug (i.e., reinstatement of a level of about 170 reinforcements versus the initial drop to about 100 reinforcements).

This result, taken alone, suggests that a sufficient number of doses in the A condition can duplicate the effects of the B condition. This prospect, considered in light of the differential effects already described, points to an obvious conclusion: the B procedure increases the rate of tolerance development so that, if relatively few injections are given, differential tolerance (B versus A) will develop. If, on the other hand, relatively more injections are given, the B and A conditions will produce comparable tolerance as in Figure 9-3.[3] There are additional implications, however.

Tolerance can be definitively determined only by a shift in the dose–response function in the direction of higher doses. Such shifts occurred for both the B and the A groups, as shown in Figure 9-3. However, the rightward shift is greater for the B group (the solid line) than for the A group (the dashed line). This result indicates that the B condition augmented the development of tolerance. (Note that tolerance is not absent in the A condition; both groups are tolerant, but the level of tolerance is greater in B than in A.) More important, these data again illustrate the crucial value of dose–response determination. In this case, testing with only a single dose (80.0 mg/kg) would have led to the conclusion that the B and A conditions were not different, when in fact they were.

This difference can be quantified by a consideration of the relevant ED_{50} values (see Chapter 8). In this case, we are concerned only with the decrease from a control level of about 170 reinforcements to 50% of that value (about 85 reinforcements). This level is indicated by the horizontal dashed line in Figure 9-3.

If we follow the horizontal line across the graph until it intersects the dose response functions, we can then read downward to determine ED_{50}s of 116.0 mg/kg for the A animals and 136.0 mg/kg for the B animals. The greater value obtained for the B group is indicative of the greater tolerance characteristic of these animals.

These results indicate that single-dose data can be very misleading, as we have repeatedly concluded before. (Recall that study of only the

80.00-mg/kg interpolated dose would have led to the conclusion that tolerance had not occurred.) We have also repeatedly concluded that the measure of pharmacologic response is a critical determinant of behavioral outcome. This latter point can be amplified by a consideration of another aspect of the results reported by Tang and Falk.

The data presented in Figure 9–4 are the response data corresponding to the reinforcements shown in Figure 9–3. The curve at the left represents the initial, pre-tolerance dose–response function; the curves at the right represent the post-tolerance functions following a series of injections given either before each of the intervening sessions (the B group—the solid curve) or after each of these sessions (the A group—the dashed curve).

The first thing to note about these data is that the ED_{50} values estimated following the development of tolerance again indicate that greater tolerance occurred in the B animals ($ED_{50} = 116.0$ mg/kg) than in the A animals ($ED_{50} = 100.0$ mg/kg). Thus, the response data concur with the reinforcement data of Figure 9–3 in indicating that greater tol-

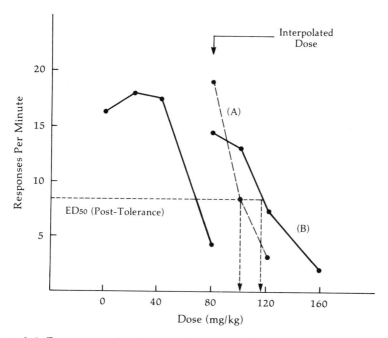

Figure 9–4. Dose–response functions as in Figure 9–3. In this case, response rates are plotted as a function of dose; numbers of reinforcements were shown in Figure 9–3. (Redrawn from Tang and Falk, 1978.)

erance occurs when injections are given before rather than after each of the intervening sessions.

However, studying the effects of only the single 80.0-mg/kg dose would have led to a very different conclusion: that the A animals, not the B, showed greater tolerance. That is, the initial response depression due to 80.0 mg/kg (to about four responses per minute) is totally erased following the development of tolerance in the A group (their level is about 19 responses per minute), whereas the B group shows only partial recovery (to a level of about 15 responses per minute).

Combining the data in Figures 9–3 and 9–4 yields the summary shown in Table 9–6.

When different measures (reinforcements versus response rate) and different modes of determination (single dose versus dose–response function) are considered, all possible conclusions about the differential effects of the B-A procedure are possible. Injections given before each intervening session can produce levels of tolerance that are greater than, less than, or the same as that produced by injections given after each session.

The fact that the single-dose comparisons generate contradictory conclusions is largely due to the fact that the post-tolerance dose–response functions in Figure 9–4 are not parallel. The function for the A treatment (the dashed curve) has a higher intercept and a steeper slope than that for the B treatment (see Figure 8–5). More to the point, the comparisons in Table 9–6 once again make it clear that single-dose data can generate very misleading conclusions.

HABITUATION AND TOLERANCE

In Chapter 7 we briefly considered the prospect that habituation (the waning of a stimulus effect) could be related to tolerance, the waning of a drug effect. (Drugs are stimuli; therefore, habituation could be involved in this waning of drug effect.) We can begin to examine this prospect by focusing on the characteristics of habituation.

Table 9–6
Degree of tolerance in B groups relative to A groups

	Reinforcements	Response Rate
Single dose (80.0 mg/kg)	Same	Less
Dose–response	Greater	Greater

THE CHARACTERISTICS OF HABITUATION

A crucial fact about habituation is that it is specific. That is, if a stimulus is repeatedly presented so that it loses its initial effect (habituation), the response will be at least partially reinstated if the stimulus or the context in which it occurs is changed.

Suppose, for example, that we study the effects of presenting a novel stimulus to a dog at rest; a stimulus such as a moderately intense noise is presented. The dog is likely to raise its head and orient toward the stimulus source; its ears may perk up, and its nostrils and pupils may dilate. As the stimulus is repeated, however, this syndrome of orienting will wane as habituation takes place. Put crudely, the novelty will wear off as boredom sets in.

But now suppose that the intensity of the noise is changed, and it is again presented. At least a partial reinstatement of the previously habituated orientation will occur. Furthermore, if the ambient illumination in the room were changed, and the noise presented again, some reinstatement would be found to occur even though the intensity of the noise had not been changed. Habituation is, in short, notably specific, both to the characteristics of the stimulus itself and to the environmental context in which it takes place.

DIFFERENTIATION OF HABITUATION AND TOLERANCE

The relationship of habituation to tolerance is summarized in Table 9–7.

When a stimulus (e.g., the moderate intensity noise, A, is presented) a behavioral change (B) will be observed. This condition is analogous to administering a drug at some intermediate dose (C). If a series of stimulus presentations intervene between A and D, then there will be a reduced effect (E) of the final presentation (D); that is, habituation will have taken place. A comparable waning of drug effect (F) can

Table 9–7

Experimental condition	Behavioral effect	Drug analog
A. Initial presentation of moderately intense stimulus	B. Change	C. Drug effect
D. Final presentation of moderately intense stimulus	E. Reduced change	F. Reduced drug effect
G. Presentation of more intense stimulus	H. Change	I. Drug effect at higher dose
J. Presentation of *less* intense stimulus	K. Change	L. (?)

occur as a consequence of repeated drug administration, as we have seen.

If a more intense stimulus (G) is now introduced, a partial or complete reinstatement of the initial effect will occur (H) because of the specificity of habituation. An analogous reinstatement due to the administration of a higher dose of drug could also occur (I) because increasing dose amounts to increasing intensity as far as the stimulus properties of drugs are concerned. That is, the reinstatement of drug effect could reflect the stimulus-specific character of habituation; in particular, the waning of drug effect (F) could reflect a waning of stimulus effect due to drug (habituation). Alternately, it could represent the rightward shift of the dose–response function that characterizes tolerance.

Whether the waning of drug effect represents habituation or tolerance cannot be determined on the basis of the effects of increased dose, because in both cases, increased dose leads to a reinstatement of behavioral change. This distinction can be made, however, on the basis of a test that involves a less intense stimulus (J). Because of the stimulus-specificity characteristic of habituation, this test will lead to reinstatement of the initial behavioral change (K). Such reinstatement cannot occur following tolerance, however.

Recall from Chapter 8 that tolerance is, by definition, a shift in the dose-response function toward higher doses. If tolerance (not apparent sensitization) has developed at a given dose level (e.g., *B* in Figure 8–2) then lower doses (e.g., less than *B*) cannot produce a reinstatement of effect.

Such reinstatement *can* occur, however. Recall that in Carey's experiment (Table 7–3), the effect of amphetamine on DRL behavior underwent a decrement but was partially reinstated by a shift to a zero dose (i.e., saline). Clearly, at least a part of this decrement can be attributed to habituation, not tolerance. That is, had the initial decrement in drug effect (responses per minute) been entirely due to tolerance, the reinstatement following administration of a zero dose (i.e., a lower stimulus intensity) could not have occurred.

HABITUATION AND ENVIRONMENTAL SPECIFICITY

Let us now examine a related idea. Might habituation be involved in the environmental specificity characteristic of behavioral tolerance?

Because it is specific to environmental context, habituation could also be a component in this environmental specificity. That is, a shift in the environment, not the stimulus itself, can lead to a reinstatement of an habituated response. There is no theoretical reason to suppose that similar processes could not apply to drug.[4]

This prospect does not, however, preclude the role that other variables may play in determining tolerance. In fact, the following factors can now be isolated:

Physiologic tolerance (e.g., enzyme induction)

Habituation

Drug-induced shifts in contingency leading to reinforcement reduction

To make matters still more complex, different behavioral procedures will be differentially sensitive to these three factors. Thus, the phenomenon of tolerance emerges as an enormously complex affair.[5]

Do not, however, allow this complexity to obscure the overriding general principle that it illustrates. Tolerance, like any other effect of a drug on behavior, is not a simple process in which the drug is administered and some particular effect irrevocably follows. If it were, tolerance would be neither environmentally specific nor procedurally specific.

These complexities can be added to the implicit list of others that we have considered in previous chapters. Such an agenda of complication naturally leads to an important question. Given the enormous complexity involved in characterizing the behavioral effects of drugs, can simple and orderly relationships between given drugs and certain behaviors ever be defined? This question is the topic of Section IV.

NOTES

1. The schedule was FI. In this case, response rates in the interval can increase, but because reinforcement is scheduled at fixed intervals, no loss of reinforcements will occur. This situation is to be contrasted with DRL, where increased response rates necessarily produce a reduction in reinforcement rate (i.e., do produce a loss).
2. The wary reader will wonder about the role of conditioned taste aversions in the B-A procedure (see Chapter 6). That is, might the injections given after ingestion produce aversions and thereby contaminate the subsequently recorded intake? The possibility is a real one. In the Carlton and Wolgin experiment, the animals were given several opportunities to eat prior to the experiment proper so that "novelty" was reduced (again see Chapter 6); internal evidence from

control animals indicated that this procedure was successful in that there were no signs of aversion. The point is nonetheless a cogent one that should be raised in considering studies involving the B-A procedure.

3. A comparable conclusion about the effects of alcohol has been drawn by LeBlanc, Gibbins, and Kalant (1973).

4. This suggestion has a formal similarity to ideas advanced by Stein (1966), by Siegel (1978a, 1978b), and by Solomon and Corbit (1974). Also, see Groves and Thompson (1970).

5. Cross-tolerance (see Chapter 8, Note 3) has, oddly, been largely neglected in studies of environmental factors in tolerance. To what extent, for example, would tolerance developed in the B-A procedure transfer to a second drug and would the degree of cross-tolerance in the A subjects be the same as that characteristic of B subjects?

Section 4
Diversity and
Classification

THE LAST CHAPTER ended on a note of complication. In particular, we saw that the physiologic factors determining tolerance can interact with environmental factors in two ways. First, the effect of physiologic factors can be contingent on the situation in which they act. Second, a drug can change environmental contingencies (produce reinforcement loss), which then exert a "feedback" effect upon the behavior to modify tolerance.

These interactions are anything but simple; to make matters still more complex, we also know that a variety of other variables can determine behavioral outcome. Let us briefly review these variables. Foremost, of course, is the particular drug chosen for study, followed by the dose studied and, much more important, the dose–response function that characterizes that drug. Equally important is the kind of behavior that is measured—motor activity, reinforced behavior, punished behavior, avoidance behavior, and so on. Other important considerations, where applicable, are the particular schedule of reinforcement involved and the nature of the behavior engendered, especially with regard to rate-dependency. We can, in fact, now construct a list of these variables:

1. Drug
2. Dose of drug
3. Dose–response function

4. Behavioral measure
5. Baseline behavior

This list is not complete, however, because still other variables, as we have seen, can affect behavior. We must also consider the possible stimulus functions of the drug—whether it is reinforcing or aversive or serves a cue function. In addition, there is the matter of drug–environment interaction so clearly exemplified in the earlier discussion of the phenomenon of tolerance. Finally, there is another variable, the particular species of animal selected for study; different species do, of course, react differently to different drugs. We can thus add three more entries to our list:

6. Stimulus functions of the drug
7. Drug–environment interaction
8. Species studied

Any one of these eight items can determine behavioral outcome, and the effects of any one can interact with those of any other to alter the net effect observed.

It is clear from this array of determinants that the effects of a drug cannot be categorized in any simple way. Similarly, differentiating among drugs can be a vastly complicated business. Indeed, the suspicion arises that, with enough experimental ingenuity, procedures could be arranged so that the effects of any one drug would appear to be identical to virtually any other. We are thus left with a profoundly troubling problem. Given the potentially dizzying diversity of behavioral outcome, how can we bring some semblance of order and simplification to the body of information concerning the behavioral effects of drugs? Must we forego organization in favor of mere itemizations of known phenomena?

Before we begin to answer these questions, we will examine briefly the kinds of problems inherent in the organization of any scientific data. Then we can approach our problem; we will do so by developing ways in which different drugs can be classified into different groups to bring order to an otherwise diffuse set of phenomena. These considerations will be the subject of Chapter 10.

The issue of classification will, in turn, set the stage for developing ways to analyze the behavioral effects of certain drugs. We will begin to examine these analytic procedures in Chapter 11.

Chapter 10

Behavioral Classification of Drugs

AS WE HAVE seen, there is an enormous potential diversity of experimental outcome. This problem is not, however, a new one. From a historical point of view, the first step in any scientific undertaking has been the development of a way to systematize information into some orderly format. Let us now examine some examples of this development.

SCIENCE AND THE PROBLEM OF DIVERSITY

The term "science" refers to, first, an organized body of knowledge and, second, the process by which that organization is achieved. The material world is replete with specific instances of objects, events, and changes; it is the business of science to bring order to this seemingly endless array of single observables.

CLASSIFICATORY SCHEMES: A HISTORICAL EXAMPLE

The scientific problem of ordering phenomena has always involved some sort of classificatory scheme that has three features: first, it is arbitrary; second, it is selective; and third, it is inevitably insufficient. The following example, which describes Mendeleev's development of the periodic table of the elements, illustrates these features.

In the mid-nineteenth century the diversity presented by the 63 elements then known was bewildering: some were gases, others were normally liquid, and others were solids; some were very hard metals, others soft; some could float on water, others were many times heavier than water; some tarnished readily, others did not; some were very reactive, others seemed to be almost inert. How could order be brought out of this diversity?

Mendeleev selected only two dimensions from this array: the chemical properties of the elements and their atomic weights. He then arbitrarily put hydrogen to one side and sorted the other 62 elements in terms of these two dimensions. A remarkable arrangement resulted. An abbreviated version of this arrangement, as it appeared in 1872, is shown in Table 10–1. (The atomic weights that he used are given in parentheses.) First, note that, by restarting the ordering process after each seventh entry, elements with similar properties fall into vertically arrayed groups, Thus, lithium (Li), sodium (Na), and potassium (K) have similar chemical properties, as do fluorine (F) and chlorine (Cl).

Table 10–1 is not the complete version developed by Mendeleev. It is, however, complete enough to make another point about the process of classification. Let us look now at the entry below boron (B) and aluminum (Al) and to the right of calcium (Ca): the next known element with an atomic weight greater than calcium was titanium (Ti) with an atomic weight of 48.0. But titanium does not have the properties of boron and aluminum; rather, it belongs with carbon (C) and silicon (Si). Accordingly, Mendeleev made a brilliant intellectual leap: He suggested that there was an as yet unknown element (a "gap") that belonged under aluminum in the table. When the remaining elements were placed in their proper position according to this assumption, each fell into place in terms of comparable properties. But then two other "gaps" appeared; Mendeleev accounted for these by assuming that they also represented unknown elements. Mendeleev went on to predict the properties of these to-be-discovered elements; as it turned out, his predictions were astonishingly accurate. For example, he predicted that the element we

Table 10–1

H	Li	Be	B	C	N	O	F
(1.0)	(7.0)	(9.4)	(11.0)	(12.0)	(14.0)	(16.0)	(19.0)
	Na	Mg	Al	Si	P	S	Cl
	(23.0)	(24.0)	(27.3)	(28.0)	(31.0)	(32.0)	(35.5)
	K	Ca	(?)	Ti			
	(39.0)	(40.0)		(48.0)			

now call germanium would have an atomic weight of "about 72" and would be ". . . a dark gray metal, density about 5.5, with a high melting point." In 1886, Winkler isolated germanium and reported that it had an atomic weight of 72.6 and was a gray metal with a density of 5.36 and a melting point of 958° C.

Mendeleev's triumph shortly ran into difficulty, as such systems inevitably do. For example, the element argon, discovered in 1894, has an atomic weight of 39.9 and would thus fall after potassium (K; 39.0) in the position occupied by calcium (Ca; 40.0) in the table. But argon is an inert gas that clearly does not share the properties of beryllium (Be) or magnesium (Mg). This and other exceptions to Mendeleev's rule set the stage for further advance. It turns out that the ordering proposed by Mendeleev *does* work if atomic number rather than atomic weight is used as the basis of the ordering.

The fact that Mendeleev's system of classification ultimately proved to be inadequate should not be surprising. Scientific statements are always provisional, and although they are sufficient at one level of analysis, they ultimately prove to be inadequate as more data accumulate. New data dictate reformulation—which itself ultimately proves to be inadequate—and another formulation is required. Thus science continues to evolve. This does not mean, however, that Mendeleev's system, for all of its arbitrariness, selectivity, and ultimate inadequacy, was useless; on the contrary, it is fair to say that the problem of understanding the degree of order that Mendeleev had delineated set the stage for the development of modern chemistry and physics.

CLASSIFICATION AND THEORY

Mendeleev's system of classification leads to an obvious question. Why should the elements arrange themselves in one particular way? There must be some underlying principle that accounts for this fact. In the case of the elements, it is the underlying atomic structure that is the basis of the classification. Thus, it is atomic number (the number of protons in the nucleus of the element)—not the atomic weights that Mendeleev used—that fully accounts for the periodic table of the elements as we know it.

But atomic theory provides an account in terms other than those used to develop the system of classification. Statements about atomic structure refer to factors other than the chemical properties of the elements or their atomic weights—to the number and arrangement of electrons, protons, and neutrons. Theory thus accounts for the order inherent in

classification but is not identical with it. Furthermore, theory cannot itself evolve if there is not an orderly classification to be accounted for
in the first place. The first step in the business of science is, then, the
development of a system of classification.

Related considerations apply to yet another example of diversity, the
enormous variety of plants and animals that are available to the most
casual observation. Today, an elaborate taxonomy brings order to this
diversity, but this has not always been so. In fact, systematic classification did not truly begin until the eighteenth century with the work of
Linnaeus.

Taxonomic classification has a tree-like character in that *kingdoms*
branch into *phyla,* each phylum divides into *classes,* and each class has
its *orders;* these orders are made up of *families;* and so on to *genus* and,
finally, *species.* This organizational system is necessarily arbitrary and is
certainly selective in that all of the characteristics of a given species are
not incorporated into it. Furthermore, there are the inevitable exceptions to the rules implied by the organization. Even at the most elementary level—the division into plant and animal kingdoms—there are
some simple multicellular organisms that are not easily classified as either plants or animals. This problem led, in the mid-nineteenth century,
to a proposal for yet another kingdom, *Protista.* But that system has its
exceptions, so that yet another kingdom, *Monera,* has been proposed to
include bacteria and certain algae. There have been, still more recently,
proposals for five- and six-kingdom systems, each based on exceptions
to the rules inherent in its predecessor.

Despite these limitations, taxonomy provides for groupings that
make it clear that the diversity of species is not simply a random assortment of possibilities. For example, chordates (e.g., humans) are obviously more like other chordates (e.g., monkeys) than they are like ar-
thropods (e.g., spiders). Similarly, sodium is more like potassium than
it is like iron in Table 10–1.

This organizational arrangement, like the periodic table, seems so
self-evident that we are likely to overlook its profound significance. The
fact that species can be meaningfully grouped leads to a theoretical
question about why they are grouped in their particular way. The question about species is not fundamentally different from the parallel question about elements.

The theoretical account of species classification brings us logically to
Darwin's conception of evolution by natural selection. There is, in the
classificatory scheme, an apparent radiation from a simple predecessor.

Darwin's theory provides for a *mechanism* by which this arrangement of individual types could occur. But the theory of natural selection operates on dimensions other than those involved in the classification. That is, the theory proposes to account for the classification but is not identical to it. Furthermore, had the classification not been available to Darwin, there would have been no basis for theory development.[1] The following two hypothetical examples illustrate this issue.

TWO HYPOTHETICAL EXAMPLES

First, suppose we had gathered together a collection of paintings by various artists. We might arrange these paintings in terms of their chronology. Were we to do so, we would find that similar paintings tend to cluster. Works by Rembrandt (1606–1669), for example, are clearly more like those by Vermeer (1632–1675) than they are like paintings by Cezanne (1839–1906); the Cezannes are more like works by Degas (1834–1917) than like the Rembrandts and Vermeers.

Such a chronological classification would leave much to be desired; Cezanne, Degas, Van Gogh (1853–1890), and Gauguin (1848–1903) were all contemporaries, yet their work is clearly disparate. We might, therefore, refine the classification to include a geographic dimension that, with the chronological, defines "schools" of painting. We would thus have a classificatory system very roughly analogous to the taxonomic groupings of plants and animals.

Our way of classifying paintings is obviously arbitrary and selective—it ignores many relevant aspects of our paintings. But does this mean it is useless? We can certainly learn more about the evolution of painting than if our collection were only a random assortment. Any system of classification is, in short, a gain over none at all, no matter how crude the system may be.

Our second hypothetical example is a quantitative rather than a qualitative one. Suppose we were to make a series of observations to which we assigned single-digit numbers. We could obtain the following:

831942287137004663 5972682

Is there some order in this sequence of observations, or is it merely a random series?

Let us address this issue by arbitrarily putting the first entry to one side (as Mendeleev did with hydrogen) and by selectively focusing on the first three digits of each successive set of four (in much the way in which Mendeleev focused on selected properties). Table 10–2 shows the arrangement we obtain.

If we now read down each of the three columns at the left of the table, we can see that there is an orderly relationship in the original sequence. (The first column is 3–2–1–0 and a repeat; the second is 1–2–3, and so on; the third is 9–8–7, and so on.) If we were to make four more observations, we could confidently state that the first three would be 1–7–7 but that the fourth would be indeterminant.

The derivation of the entries in Table 10–2 is arbitrary and is certainly selective in that it ignores both the initial value (8) and the fourth digit in each set. But those insufficiencies do not mean that there is no gain over assuming that the original sequence is a meaninglessly random one. Furthermore, we might be able to develop a theory about the phenomena from which the numbers are derived. Such a theory would have to account, of course, for the particular sequence of values uncovered. Such a theory might or might not be successful, but we certainly could not have undertaken theorization if we did not have orderly data in the first place.

There are two other lessons to be drawn from this example. First, the discovery of order by the development of classification requires a large body of data. We could not have "cracked the code" involved in the number sequence (Table 10–2) if we had had only a few entries. Similarly, Mendeleev obviously could not have developed his table if he had had only a few elements to work with.

Second, it would have been impossible to develop the classification shown in Table 10–2 if the numbers were not themselves reliable ones, for if they were not, the systematic relations apparent in the table could not have been found. Similarly, Mendeleev could not have developed his table if the determination of atomic weights had not been reliable. If the value for sodium (Na), for example, was sometimes found to be

Table 10–2

Initial Digit	First Three Digits of Set			Fourth Digit of Set
8	3	1	9	4
	2	2	8	7
	1	3	7	0
	0	4	6	6
	3	5	9	7
	2	6	8	2

23 and sometimes 24, or the value for phosphorus (P) was sometimes determined to be 31 but to be 32 at other times, Mendeleev could not have used atomic weight to reliably discriminate sodium from magnesium (Mg) or phosphorus from sulfur (S).

A RUDIMENTARY DRUG CLASSIFICATION

Classification is, as we have just seen, arbitrary, selective, and incomplete. But no matter how crude it may be, it has the potential to tell us more than a purely random assortment ever can. We have also seen that classification requires an accumulation of a substantial body of information that is reliable.

This last consideration means that, when we approach the problem of classifying drugs, we will have to follow a path that is dictated by the quantity and reliability of the available information. The preliminary classification offered by Dews and DeWeese (1977) is a case in point.

Dews and DeWeese have surveyed the available literature with respect to these two criteria: a very large quantity of data that is sufficiently reliable to permit classification. Because of these severe constraints, the result is restricted to three drugs and four procedures.

An adaptation of the classification developed by Dews and DeWeese is given in Table 10–3. The (+) entries indicate an increase in overall responding, (−) entries indicate a decrease, and (0) entries indicate no consistent effect. The first entry refers to the lowest dose range with a clear effect; the second entry indicates the effect of dose in the middle range; and the effects of high doses, indicated by the third entry, generally decrease behavior. The dose–response curves summarized in this way are thus not quantitative (in mg). Rather, the table provides a shorthand method of showing the effects seen in the lower, middle, and upper portions of the effective dose range of each drug.

The table indicates that low doses of pentobarbital increase FI responding (entry 1) but that middle and high doses decrease it. In contrast, FR responding (entry 2) is increased by a wider range of doses that includes the midrange doses that decrease FI responding (compare the middle symbols in entries 1 and 2). Entry 3 indicates that pentobarbital decreases discriminated avoidance responding at all dose levels (low, medium, and high). Such an entry is meant to imply a monotonic, decreasing dose–response function (decrease in the middle range that is greater than at low doses but less than that characteristic of high

Table 10–3

Procedure	Drug Class		
	I. Pentobarbital	*II. Amphetamine*	*III. Chlorpromazine*
FI	1. (+)(−)(−)	5. (+)(+)(−)	9. (−)(−)(−)
FR	2. (+)(+)(−)	6. (0) (−)(−)	10. (−)(−)(−)
Nondiscriminated avoidance	3. (−)(−)(−)	7. (+)(+)(−)	11. (−)(−)(−)
Punishment	4. (+)(+)(−)	8. (0) (0) (0)	12. (−)(−)(−)

Modified from Dews and DeWeese, 1977.

doses). Analogously, a (+) (−) indicates biphasic dose–response curves like those discussed in Chapter 3 (see Figure 3–2).

The table also tells us that pentobarbital increases punished responding, that it will do so at doses that decrease FI responding (the middle dose range), and that neither amphetamine nor chlorpromazine has this property. Similarly, pentobarbital uniquely increases FR responding (compare entry 2 with entries 6 and 10).

Entry 5 indicates that amphetamine has a biphasic effect on FI responding and that it increases such responding in the low dose range but has no effect on FR responding in this range (entry 6). Amphetamine also has an effect on nondiscriminated avoidance, which parallels its effect on FI, but has no consistent effect on punished responding.

Finally, there is chlorpromazine, a drug that differs from the others in that it produces dose-dependent decrements in responding in all four procedures.

The arrangement in Table 10–3 is a rudimentary first step toward classification. Rudimentary as it is, however, it does generate several potentially important questions.

DEFINITION OF CLASSES

It may be that pentobarbital, amphetamine, and chlorpromazine define larger classes (Classes I, II, and III) into which other drugs will fall. Pentobarbital, for example, shares many of the properties of a larger group, as we shall see in Chapter 12; it remains to be seen whether all of these will conform to the pattern of Class I. Similarly, chlorpromazine shares many of the properties of yet another large group (see Chapter 13). Will all of these conform to the Class III pattern?

One value of a classificatory system is that it sets the boundaries for further classification. Only further research can tell us the extent to which Table 10–3 will prove to be useful. We can surely anticipate that other classes will evolve as exceptions to the rules implicit in Table 10–3 emerge. On the other hand, it is not extravagant to suppose that relatively few classes will ultimately characterize all behaviorally active drugs.

CHARACTERISTICS OF CLASSES

As shown in Table 10–3, pentobarbital (which may define Class I) is the only drug that increases both FR and punished responding. This fact naturally leads us to ask whether there is a relationship underlying this parallel in two seemingly very different behaviors. Alternatively, we can ask why it is that chlorpromazine (Class III) uniquely decreases responding, regardless of schedule. (The answer cannot simply be that it is a depressant; pentobarbital is a depressant too.) Similarly, we can wonder why it is that amphetamine (Class II) is uniquely ineffective in altering punished responding.

We do not yet know what the answers to those questions might be. This is not the point in the present context, however; rather, it is that these questions could not have been asked if we did not have the classification before us.

AN ALTERNATIVE MODE OF CLASSIFICATION

The classification we have been considering is entirely empirical in the sense that it is dictated by the quantity and quality of available information. We can now consider another mode of classification, one that is empirical in another sense.

As it happens, a large body of behavioral information has grown up around a few classes of drugs. This classification is based on the *clinical* use of these drugs, not solely on the available laboratory information (as in Table 10–3). A brief digression will clarify why there has been this particular accumulation of data.

PHARMACOLOGY AND MEDICINE; BEHAVIORAL PHARMACOLOGY AND PSYCHIATRY

It is a matter of historical fact that pharmacology has evolved as a crucial adjunct to medicine. Thus, emphasis within the field of pharmacology has been placed on elucidating the properties of those drugs having demonstrable clinical use. As a result, caffeine, for example, receives relatively little discussion in pharmacology texts, whereas morphine receives relatively much more. Although it is certainly true that caffeine use (in coffee, tea, and colas) is far more extensive than the use of morphine, emphasis is on the latter because of its relatively greater clinical significance.

Behavioral pharmacology is a subdiscipline of pharmacology; just as pharmacology is an adjunct to medicine, behavioral pharmacology has evolved as an adjunct to a subdiscipline of medicine: psychiatry. Psychiatry is primarily concerned with the management of clinically disordered behavior, so-called psychopathology. Furthermore, there can be no doubt that a major means of effecting such management is by the administration of drugs. There has been, therefore, a natural union of emphasis in psychiatry and behavioral pharmacology: both focus on the behavioral effects of drugs. Furthermore, this focus has been on a few drugs, selected because of their psychiatric relevance.

This is not to say, however, that this state of affairs is necessarily the way things should be. There is no reason why caffeine or nicotine, for example, could not form an important aspect of behavioral drug characterization, We have, in fact, already noted (Table 10–3) the potential power of a classification devoid of any particular medical or psychiatric emphasis. But the fact remains that, in behavioral pharmacology, there has been a selective emphasis on drugs of psychiatric relevance; in this area of psychiatric relevance there has been a massive accumulation of data focused on only three groups of drugs and on a single drug, lithium.

The first group is the **anxiolytics** (or antianxiety drugs), drugs useful in the clinical management of anxiety (to be discussed in Chapter 12); the second group includes the **neuroleptics**, drugs useful in the clinical management of psychosis in general and schizophrenia in particular (Chapter 13); the third group (Chapter 14) includes the **antidepressants,** drugs that are useful in managing clinical depression; **lithium,** a drug that is useful in managing mania, will also be discussed in chapter 14.

CLINICAL CLASSIFICATION AND THE ANALYSIS OF MECHANISM

We have, then, a classification based on demonstrable clinical use. For example, one group of drugs that is of unquestionable efficacy in the management of clinical anxiety is the anxiolytics. There is, of course, a much larger group that is not efficacious. Thus, clinical use provides us with an elementary system of classification—anxiolytics and non-anxiolytics.

Given this, we can turn to the question that classification always engenders. Why is it that these particular drugs cluster in the way that they do? That is, why is it that some drugs fall into one class and other drugs fall into others?

We will need to address three issues if we are to develop an answer to this question.

DIAGNOSTIC CLASSIFICATION AS BEHAVIOR

The first issue relates to the bases on which the drugs we are considering are prescribed in the first place. Prescription is based on a diagnosis, and as we shall see, these diagnoses are intrinsically behavioral in nature.

Diagnoses of anxiety, psychosis, or depression are necessarily based on behavior of three types:

1. Verbal behavior of the patient: for example, "I feel frightened all the time" (anxiety); "Nothing seems worthwhile" (depression); "I hear the voice of my dead brother all the time" (psychosis—i.e., schizophrenia).
2. Verbal behavior of others: for example, friends, family, physician, or nurses may report that the patient "looks anxious," "seems depressed," or talks in a "crazy" way.[2]
3. Motor behavior of the patient: for example, the anxious patient may "fidget"; the psychotic may engage in obviously bizarre behavior. (Note that these behaviors are generally reported by others or by the patient.)

These examples vastly oversimplify the generality and complexity of data that go into an actual psychiatric diagnosis; we will be considering more detailed case histories in later chapters.[3] For the moment, however, we need only note one salient point: The diagnoses we are considering are based on behavioral indices, not on laboratory test results (e.g., low blood sugar in diabetics or X-ray visualization of tumors in cancer).

CLINICAL DRUG RESPONSE AS BEHAVIOR

The second issue focuses on the changes produced by the different drugs we are considering. These changes are, of course, also based on verbal behaviors or reports of change in motor behavior (e.g., "I don't feel anxious anymore"; "The patient is no longer pacing the ward, wringing his hands and complaining that his thoughts are controlled by others"). Thus, the clinical drug responses that form the basis of the classification are themselves behavioral.

There is no reason whatsoever for supposing that these drug-induced changes in behavior are immune to the complex kinds of determination described in previous chapters. Indeed, clinical drug responses of the type considered here are notorious for their variability and interaction with a broad range of variables.[4] Despite this complexity, however, the fact of the matter is that a few drugs *do* selectively reduce anxiety and most other drugs do not; a few *do* ameliorate depression and most others do not; a few *do* control psychotic symptoms and most others do not. Furthermore, those that are useful in the management of anxiety are not generally useful in managing depression or psychosis; the antidepressants are not generally useful in reducing anxiety or managing psychosis; the neuroleptics are not generally useful in managing anxiety or depression. Thus, a small number of drugs can be sorted into relatively distinct classes on the basis of the behavioral changes they produce.[5]

THE NEED FOR LABORATORY ANALYSIS

Why is it that certain drugs can be classified as anxiolytic, neuroleptic, or antidepressant? The answer lies in the physiologic-biochemical effects of these drugs. The ultimate question, then, is a more basic one: What are the underlying processes that account for the fact that there is a classification at all?

For example, why do certain elements "cluster" as they do in the periodic table? A part of the answer could be given in terms of electron configuration: The configurations for the elements in Mendeleev's first group—lithium, sodium, and potassium—are 2–1, 1–8–1, and 2–8–8–1, respectively. The configurations for the elements in his second group—beryllium, magnesium, and calcium—are 2–2, 2–8–2, 2–8–8–2, respectively. A difference between the first and second groups is that elements in the first have a single electron in their outer shells, whereas those in the second group have two. We can thus specify a mechanism that accounts for the fact that certain elements fall into a certain class, other elements fall into another class, and so on. But can we specify analogous mechanisms that will account for the clinical classification we are considering here? That is, can we specify physiologic-biochemical effects shared by all anxiolytics but not by other drugs in a way that would be analogous to the electron configurations we just discussed? Can we similarly specify other effects shared by the antidepressants to account for the fact that they are grouped as they are? Can we specify effects shared by the neuroleptics to account for their communality of clinical action?[6]

Unfortunately, our approach to such questions about mechanism will immediately reveal a serious problem. Consider, as an example, the drug group labeled "anticholinergic" (analogous to "anxiolytic"). Two facts are relevant: First, we know that a number of drugs have one set of clinical effects in common; they thus fall into a class of their own. It turns out that, second, all of these drugs can be shown to attenuate the actions of acetylcholine (ACH; see Chapter 3). (They are thus called anticholinergics.) More to the point, their common mechanism of action is the ACH attenuation they all produce. It is this communality (analogous to electron configuration) that accounts for the grouping.

However, when we say that a drug blocks the action of ACH, we are relying on facts that derive from a variety of surgical and biochemical procedures that cannot be undertaken in humans. That is, this elucidation of mechanism involves a laboratory analysis.

But how can we generate a parallel laboratory analysis of the classification we are considering? We will need laboratory models of the different clinical drug responses that produce the different classifications. We will begin to consider the problem of developing such models in the following chapter.

NOTES

1. The foregoing material has been primarily derived from discussions in Jaffee (1957), Kieffer (1971), and Bronowski (1973).
2. These verbal reports may be formalized in the form of rating scales or diagnostic checklists. They are, nonetheless, instances of verbal behavior.
3. The behaviors that go into diagnosis are determined by complex factors and are variable over time. As a result, the reliability of psychiatric diagnosis tends to be relatively low.
4. For example, the clinical response to antianxiety drugs has been shown to vary with the following:

   Sex of patient
   Marital status of patient
   Patient's expectation about drug treatment
   Presence of side-effects (primarily sedation)
   Physician's expectation about prognosis

[See Rickels, Downing, and Winokur (1978).]

5. The classification is statistical in nature. That is, responses of only two patients given the same drug could be expected to differ because of the complexities involved in drug-induced behavioral change. On the other hand, for large numbers of patients, the clinical classification discussed here emerges.

6. It is vitally important to recognize that, even if we could specify a mechanism for one class of drugs, this fact alone could not conceivably account for *all* of the behavioral effects of that class. As we have seen in previous chapters, the actions of drugs are determined by multiple factors so that behavioral outcome cannot be conceptualized as inhering solely in the physiologic-biochemical effects of the drug itself.

Chapter 11

Classification, Analysis and Laboratory Models

CHAPTER 10 ENDED with a discussion of a mode of classification based on demonstrable clinical use. We then raised a question about mechanism. What are the basic properties of different drugs that generate the classification? That is, what are the mechanisms that allow some drugs to be classed as anxiolytic, others as antidepressant, and so on? Unfortunately, the necessary analysis usually cannot be undertaken at a clinical level in humans. We therefore need laboratory models.

THE NEED FOR LABORATORY MODELS OF CLINICAL DRUG RESPONSE

The classification we are considering is based on different clinical drug responses (i.e., reports of symptom reduction produced by different classes of drugs). This means that certain clinical phenomena are modified by certain drugs. We want to elucidate the mechanisms that produce this clinical drug response. Note that we are focusing our attention on the clinical drug response, not on the clinical phenomenon itself. Thus, in the case of the anxiolytics, for example, our primary concern is not with the phenomenon of anxiety per se but with the analysis of the reduction in anxiety due to drug.

However, as noted at the end of the last chapter, such analyses are very likely to be impossible because the appropriate experimental procedures cannot be carried out in humans. The following example amplifies the nature of the problem. Suppose that we had a group of drugs that produced blood pressure reductions in hypertensive patients. We would also find that this same class of drugs produced blood pressure reductions in laboratory animals. Given that fact, we could use the laboratory animals to analyze the physiologic mechanisms underlying the drug response. We would then find that some of the drugs in question reduce blood pressure because they produce vasodilation (i.e., they enlarge blood vessels so that the net pressure in the "hydraulic" circulatory system is less). We might then find that this dilation occurs because the drugs antagonize the actions of naturally occurring substances that normally act to constrict blood vessels. As a moment's reflection will indicate, however, most of the surgical, biochemical, and other physiologic interventions required for such an analysis could not be undertaken in humans. The analysis requires a laboratory model of the clinical drug response.

As we shall see, the analysis of behavioral change due to drug requires procedures that are analogous to the one used in the analysis of blood pressure reduction. Note, however, that our problem is still more complex because our clinical measures cannot be identical to our laboratory measures. (In contrast, blood pressure could be used in both the clinic and the laboratory in the previous example.) In our case, the behavioral changes are reported reductions in the symptoms of anxiety, schizophrenia, depression, or mania, and there are simply no changes in laboratory behavior that can be simply and directly related to these drug effects. What, for example, is the behavior of a laboratory rat made "less anxious," "less depressed," or "less schizophrenic" by drug?

Thus, the laboratory behavior used in our model will not necessarily mirror the clinical phenomenon in question. This is not our objective, however; rather, our goal is to isolate a laboratory drug response that will have characteristics that will permit us to plausibly say that the laboratory drug response is a suitable model for the analysis of the corresponding clinical drug response. How, then, can we develop such a model?

DEVELOPING A MODEL OF CLINICAL DRUG RESPONSE

We need some laboratory behavior with which the fact of clinical classification can be analyzed. But we know that the behavioral effects of drug can vary widely as a consequence of a variety of other interacting variables. How, then, are we to isolate a single behavior that can then serve us as a basis for analysis?

To answer this question, we will select some behavioral index of drug action to be studied in the laboratory and then evaluate the extent to which this laboratory model mirrors the characteristics of a clinical drug response. That is, we will examine the degree to which the characteristics of a laboratory drug response parallel those of a clinical drug response.

The selection of the laboratory behavior to be studied will not, of course, be made at random; there are valuable leads in the available literature, as we shall see in subsequent chapters. For the moment, however, we will focus on the characteristics of the clinical drug response that can be used to evaluate the adequacy of a particular model. But what are these characteristics? We will begin to answer this question by identifying four characteristics that may apply to any clinical drug response.[1]

First, we know that certain drugs will produce a given clinical effect, whereas most others will not. Second, we know that, among those that do produce the effect, different drugs will have different potencies in doing so. Third, the effects of a drug may occur rapidly, or full development of an effect may require a substantial period of chronic medication; chronic medication may lead to the development of tolerance in other instances. Finally, some drug effects are augmented (or antagonized) by other treatments.

Now suppose that we have selected some behavioral response to drug in the hope that it will provide us with a useful model of some clinical drug response. If that laboratory drug response is to be a useful model, it should have the following characteristics:

1. If the clinical drug response is produced by only a few drugs and not by others, then the laboratory response should be produced by those few and not by others.
2. If different clinically effective drugs have different potencies, then the same relative potencies should hold in the case of the laboratory response.
3. If a clinical response is characterized by rapid (or delayed) onset and tolerance does not occur (or does occur), then the laboratory response should occur rapidly (or be delayed) and should not show tolerance (or tolerate).
4. If the clinical response is antagonized (or augmented) by some auxil-

lary treatment, then the laboratory response should also be antagonized (or augmented) by the same treatment.

The relationship between clinical response and laboratory response
can be further clarified by imagining that, first, the clinical response is
determined by a hypothetical set of factors and that a second hypothetical set determines the laboratory response. If a number of factors are
common to both sets, then the characteristics of the two responses (clinical and laboratory) should be parallel. Conversely, to the extent that
they do not share determining factors, their characteristics will not be
parallel. Thus, the extent to which the characteristics of a clinical response are mirrored in those of a laboratory response can be used as
a guide to the adequacy of the latter as a model of the former.

CRITERIA FOR LABORATORY MODELS

The general relationships we have been considering provide a set of
criteria by which the adequacy of a laboratory model can be evaluated.
We will consider some of the details of these criteria in the remainder
of this chapter and then turn to specific applications of the criteria in
Section V.

CRITERION A: DIFFERENTIATION, FALSE POSITIVES, AND
FALSE NEGATIVES

The basis of the clinical classification discussed in Chapter 10 is the fact
that some drugs produce a change in particular behaviors, whereas other
drugs do not. We have already seen that, if the factors controlling behavioral change in our model include those determining clinical response, then the model should differentiate drugs just as the clinical
drug response does. As more and more factors are common to these two,
the greater will be the degree of the parallelism in effect. We can sche-
matize a somewhat more elaborate version of this relationship by the
arrangement in Table 11–1.

As we have repeatedly seen, all drugs have multiple effects. One of
these effects may be the reduction in symptoms that defines a particular
class; other effects are secondary to this activity (so-called
"side-effects"). We can call these drugs *Type I*. Other drugs may not produce symptom reduction but can produce the same secondary effects
as those of Type I drugs; these are labeled *Type II* in the table. Still other
drugs, *Type III*, have effects of their own, but these include neither symptom reduction nor the secondary effects of Type I and Type II.

Table 11–1

Drug Type	Clinical Effects	Positive Response in Model
I	Symptom reduction + secondary effects	Yes
II	Secondary effects only	No
III	Neither symptom reduction nor secondary effects	No

If the particular laboratory measure chosen is to be a candidate as a model, it should, at the very least, show the pattern of positive responses listed at the right of Table 11–1. That is, the model should be selectively sensitive to Type I drugs. Looked at another way, it should differentiate drugs in the same way that the clinical response (symptom reduction) differentiates them.

There are two other implications of the table that we should consider. The first of these pertains to the difference between Type I and Type II drugs. As we shall find in later chapters, a number of drugs can produce the secondary effects of a clinically efficacious drug without themselves being efficacious. This fact means that the symptom reduction characteristic of some drugs cannot be attributed to these secondary effects; if they could, all drugs having secondary effects would be efficacious. Antidepressants (Type I), for example, produce anticholinergic effects similar to those produced by atropine or scopolamine. It could be supposed that antidepressant activity is due to anticholinergic activity. But if this were true, atropine and scopolamine would be effective antidepressants—which they very definitely are not. They are, therefore, Type II drugs with regard to reduction in the symptoms of depression.

More directly pertinent to the business of model development is the fact that an insensitivity of the model to Type II drugs means that the laboratory drug response is not based on secondary effects. This leads directly to the second implication: As previously discussed, both false positives and false negatives can occur when laboratory drug response and clinical drug response are compared. Consider Table 11–2.

Table 11–2

Clinical Change	Positive Laboratory Response	
	No	*Yes*
Yes (Type I)	1	2
No (Types I and II)	3	4

Ideally, all drugs should fall into either group 2 or group 3. But such an outcome is very unlikely because it could occur only if there were a perfect relationship between the clinical drug response (behavioral change in humans) and our model (behavioral change in a laboratory animal). We can, therefore, expect both false negatives (group 1) and false positives (group 4). That is, the laboratory measure may fail to detect a truly efficacious drug—the negative response of the model is false (group 1)—or it may generate a positive response to a drug lacking efficacy—the positive response is false (group 4).

Although it is unrealistic to expect that any model will be fully free of both false positives and false negatives, the extent to which this ideal is approached can be used as a guide to evaluating a model. The extent to which the model leads to categorization into groups 2 and 3, but not into groups 1 and 4, can predict how useful the model will be in analyzing the relevant clinical drug response.[2]

CRITERION B: POTENCY RELATIONS

We have thus far considered a basic criterion for any model of clinical drug response: it should differentiate clinically effective drugs from ineffective ones. We can now turn to a more refined version of the same idea: the model should detect the potencies of different drugs in a way that is directly related to the clinical potencies of these same drugs.

Suppose we know that each of five drugs, A through E, is clinically effective (they all reduce anxiety, say). Further suppose that we have an estimate of the potencies of these different drugs in clinical use. That is, we know the dose of Drug A that will produce a given level of symptom control (e.g., anxiety reduction), the dose of Drug B that will produce this same level of control, and so on. We will call these values their **clinical potencies.**

Now suppose that the model that we are trying to construct will differentiate clinically active from inactive drugs in terms of some response of the model (Criterion A)—clinically active drugs produce the response; inactive ones do not. We can now calculate the potency of each of these *active* drugs in terms of their MED, ED_{50}, or some other single value estimating potency. That is, we can obtain a single value that tells us the dose of Drug A that is required to produce a given level of positive response, the dose of Drug B that is required, and so on. We can call these values **laboratory potencies.** We now have a pair of values for each drug: the clinical potency and the laboratory potency.

To the extent that the factors controlling clinical and laboratory responses are shared, we can expect that drugs with higher clinical potency will be more potent in producing a response in the model, whereas those with lower clinical potency will have a relatively lower laboratory potency. Put another way, the idea of a model assumes that there are factors that control clinical response and that some of these factors also control laboratory response; the extent to which this assumption is true will be indicated by the extent to which laboratory potencies parallel clinical potencies. On the other hand, if very few factors are common to the two classes of response (those recorded in the clinic and those recorded in the laboratory), there will then be little relation between the two sets of potencies.

Consider the hypothetical data in Table 11–3. The drugs, all of which are clinically active, are arranged in terms of increasing potency in the first column; the clinical doses are themselves given in the second column. (Recall that a higher dose means that the drug is less potent.) The parenthetical values after each dose give the rank ordering of potencies.

The values in the third column are hypothetical doses (MEDs, $ED_{50}s$ or some other single-value estimate) for Drugs A through E for one laboratory measure, (I). It is clear that the relationship of potencies is perfect: The more potent a drug in the clinic, the more potent it is in the laboratory model. But now consider the data obtained with another laboratory measure, (II), in the column at the far right. In this case, the relationship is quite poor.

The relative strength of these relationships can be seen in terms of the rank orders of potencies given in parentheses. The ordering of clinical potencies (1 through 5 for Drugs A through E) is perfectly parallel to that for Measure I; there are no reversals of position. In contrast, the data obtained with Measure II show only a very irregular relationship to the corresponding clinical potencies. Thus, Measure I provides a substantially better model of clinical drug response than that supplied by Measure II.

Table 11–3

Clinically Active Drugs	Clinical Dose (mg)	Laboratory Measure I	Dose (mg)/(kg) Measure II
A	100 (5)	10 (5)	4 (3)
B	75 (4)	8 (4)	10 (5)
C	50 (3)	4 (3)	1 (1)
D	20 (2)	3 (2)	8 (4)
E	5 (1)	1 (1)	3 (2)

There are several ways of portraying the relationships given in Table 11–3. One of these is in graphic form, as shown in Figure 11–1. The values in the top panel of the figure show the relationship of clinical dose to laboratory dose for Measure I; comparable values for Measure II are shown at the bottom. Clearly, the results for Measure I are characterized by an orderly relationship to clinical dose, whereas those for Measure II are not.

Rather than a graphic presentation, a numerical index can be used

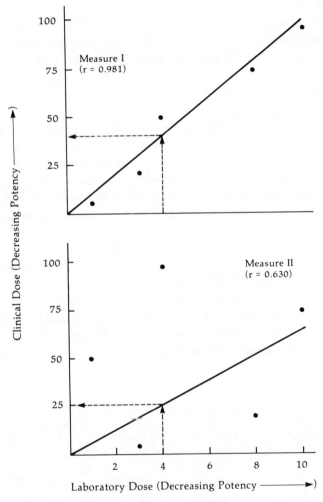

Figure 11–1. Graphic representations of the relationships between laboratory dose and clinical dose for Measure I (top) and for Measure II (bottom).

to summarize these relationships. The most commonly used value is a **correlation coefficient** (or, strictly speaking, a Pearson product–moment correlation). The details of computation are not necessary here; suffice it to say that the correlation coefficient (symbolized as r) can range from 1.00 (indicating a perfect relationship) to zero (indicating no relationship) down to -1.00 (indicating a perfect inverse relationship). As would be expected, this index is nearly perfect in the case of Measure I ($r = 0.981$) and much lower in the case of Measure II ($r = 0.630$).

Consideration of these two values of r highlights an important feature of the correlation coefficient. The fact of the matter is that correlation coefficients in the middle range of values can be quite deceptive. Let us make some detailed comparisons of the data in Figure 11–1 to clarify the issue.

For Measure I, it is clear that the clinical dose of a given drug could be rather accurately predicted on the basis of its laboratory dose. Suppose, for example, that we select the laboratory dose for Drug C obtained from Measure I (4.0 mg; see Table 11–3). We can then project a line from this value on the abscissa to the point at which it intersects the line describing the relationship and then project this value onto the ordinate. As indicated by the dashed arrows in the figure, we obtain a value of about 41.0 mg, which compares favorably with the actual value of 50.0 mg in Table 11–3. But now consider Drug A and Measure II: The laboratory dose is again 4.0 mg/kg, but the predicted clinical dose is about 25.0 mg, a value that is very different from the true clinical value of 100.0 mg.[3]

What is needed is some index of the efficiency of the model in predicting clinical dose. One such index (from Guildford, 1936) is provided by the equation

$$100 \left(1 - \sqrt{1 - r^2}\right)$$

The values obtained from this equation, called the **index of forecasting efficiency,** or **IFE,** provide a direct estimate of the percentage reduction of errors in prediction for a given value of r. The relationship of IFE to r is given in Figure 11–2.[4]

The relationship in the figure indicates that, with increasing values of r, forecasting efficiency increases very little below the middle of the range of values. In terms of our example, an r of 0.63 (for measure II) has an IFE of about 22%. Thus, the IFE for Measure I (80%) is about *four* times greater than that for Measure II, even though the r for Mea-

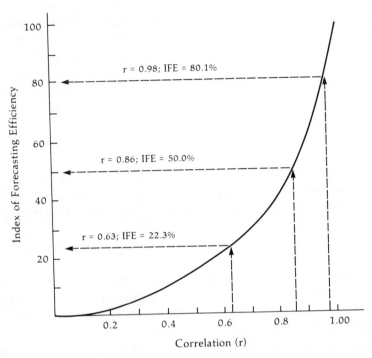

Figure 11–2. Relationship of the correlation coefficient *(r)* to the Index of Forecasting Efficiency (IFE). The IFEs corresponding to selected values of *r* are indicated by the arrows.

sure I is only about one and one-half times greater than that for Measure II (0.981 versus 0.630). Looked at in this way, one half of a perfect correlation (r = 1.000, IFE = 100%) is 0.866 (IFE = 50%), not 0.500 (IFE = 13%).

In general, for evaluation of laboratory models in terms of their efficiency in predicting the clinical potencies of different drugs, the IFE provides a much more useful guide than does the value of *r* itself.

CRITERION C: TEMPORAL CHARACTERISTICS

A clinical drug response can be characterized by, first, the temporal nature of the onset of drug activity and, second, the development of tolerance in the course of repeated drug administration.

As far as the first kind of temporal characteristic is concerned, the onset of clinical activity may be quite rapid or may require a substantial period of medication before a clear drug response appears. In this regard, the anxiolytics that we will consider in the next chapter are to be contrasted with the neuroleptics (Chapter 13) and with the antidepressants and lithium (Chapter 14); onset of activity following anxiolytic medication occurs in minutes, whereas clinical response may require weeks in the other cases.

The degree of communality between a model and a clinical drug response can also be evaluated by considering the temporal characteristics of a positive response in the model: if clinical response is rapid, laboratory response should be rapid, and if clinical activity is delayed, laboratory response should be delayed.

Similar considerations apply to the second temporal factor, tolerance. If clinical response wanes despite continued medication, then tolerance should also be characteristic of the laboratory response and vice versa. Of particular importance in this context is the fact that the clinical effects of a drug may show differential tolerance. That is, of the several clinical drug effects initially obtained, some may wane whereas others are maintained. The neuroleptics, for example, produce a variety of initial effects, two of which are particularly noteworthy. One of these is, of course, the decrement in schizophrenic behaviors for which the drugs are prescribed in the first place; a secondary effect involves disturbances of motor function that are collectively called the *extrapyramidal syndrome,* or EPS (see Chapter 13). Differential tolerance to neuroleptic activity is evident in the waning of EPS despite a maintenance of symptom control during the course of chronic medication. Such instances of differential tolerance can provide important clues for analyzing clinical drug response, as we shall see.

CRITERION D: DRUG INTERACTIONS

The clinical response obtained with some of the drugs we will be considering are either antagonized or potentiated by the concurrent activity of other drugs. Furthermore, such antagonism or synergism may be selective in that some, but not all, of the effects of the drug can be altered by yet another drug. EPS due to neuroleptics, for example, can be antagonized by other drugs (anti-EPS medications) that do not themselves antagonize the primary clinical drug response (reduction of schizophrenic symptoms).

CRITERION E: EVALUATION IN HUMANS

Our final criterion, one that we have not considered before, follows from the preceding four. Suppose that all of the criteria, A through D, just discussed can be reasonably well met. Thus, many of the factors controlling the clinical drug response apparently are shared by the laboratory response. But if this implication is correct, it should be possible to show explicitly that the drug-induced behavioral change seen in the laboratory can also be obtained when the test species is human. That is, drug administration in human subjects following exposure to whatever behavioral procedure has been adopted should yield results qualitatively similar to those obtained in laboratory animals.

This step in the evaluation of laboratory models is an important, albeit largely neglected one. After all, if clinical and laboratory drug responses do truly share factors, then the laboratory drug response should be obtainable in humans.

Note that our concern is with the laboratory drug response, not simply with a replication of the clinical drug response itself. If, for example, we were to obtain some behavioral effect of the anxiolytics in laboratory animals, and if this effect were to satisfy Criteria A through D, then we would want to know if the characteristics of this effect also obtain in humans. We are not at this point interested in again showing that the anxiolytics reduce the clinical signs of anxiety.

It may, of course, not be possible to impose behavioral procedures that are identical to those used in laboratory animals because of the ethical constraints that led to the use of laboratory models in the first place. It should, nonetheless, be possible to develop some approximation of the animal procedure that is applicable to humans and, at the very least, to show a rough parallelism of drug effect in these two species. If this cannot be done, the applicability of a model to the clinical drug response will be suspect.

EMPIRICAL VALIDITY VERSUS FACE VALIDITY

In considering the criteria just discussed, we are concerned with the validity of models as laboratory representations of clinical drug response. To the extent that the various criteria are met, we can say that the model is **empirically valid.** That is, the parallelism of effect between clinical and laboratory response has been experimentally determined and assessed. In other words, as more criteria are met to a greater and greater extent, it becomes progressively more reasonable to suppose that a greater number of the factors that determine clinical drug response also determine laboratory drug response. There is, then, a substantial communality in the determination of the two.

But there is a second kind of validity, one that has historically been involved in the kinds of models we are considering. It is called **face validity.** In this usage, "face" means that the two behaviors—clinical and laboratory—appear to be the same. There is, therefore, validity to the model "on the face of it."

There are at least two major problems with this view of validity. In the first place, it carries with it the idea that, in studies of aberrant clinical behavior, the laboratory behavior observed should be comparably aberrant. For example, in studies involving the effects of anxiolytics, the laboratory animals used in the model should somehow *look* anxious.

But this implication confuses a model of a clinical phenomenon with a model of clinical drug response—and these are not the same, as we have seen. There is, in fact, no reason why the behavior seen in the laboratory should necessarily appear to be comparable to that seen clinically. A particular instance of laboratory behavior could meet all of the criteria discussed without an obvious resemblance of that behavior to the aberrant behavior seen in the clinic. Thus, the issue lies not in the nature of appearances but in the degree of demonstrable parallelism contained in the criteria that underlie empirical validation.

The second problem with reliance on face validity is an implication that the laboratory procedure used for the model should "look like" one that would produce a comparable effect in the clinic. Subjecting an animal to electric shock, for example, is an apparently anxiety-provoking procedure. As we have seen, however, shock presentation can either suppress behavior or maintain it (see Note 4, Chapter 6), depending on the particulars of the experimental situation. Appearances can be deceiving.

Both variants of face validity—the appearance of the behavior and the procedure that controls it—involve a reliance on anthropomorphic judgment in determining the extent of validity. In this view, a rat that *looks* anxious or a procedure that *looks* as if it should engender anxiety thus consitutes a valid model for the analysis of anxiolytic activity in the clinic. It is not clear, however, just how these judgments are to be evaluated: Precisely what does an anxious rat actually look like? Why should it look like an anxious human? Just what does an anxious snail look like? (Should such species be dismissed from consideration?) Why should a procedure that appears to be anxiety-provoking to humans also induce anxiety in laboratory animals? The list of questions can obviously be lengthened.

Face validity is a pervasive idea, probably becasue we humans take the view that all other species should somehow represent us. A model should not, however, be rejected simply because face validity is lacking. There is no reason why the behavior of a snail, for example, could not provide an entirely useful, empirically validated model—even though snails do not do much of anything resembling human activity. More to the point, evaluation of a model should never rest solely on its face validity in the absence of empirical validation. Although this point seems self-evident, the rule has not uniformly been followed, often with unfortunate consequences for the elucidation of phenomena. We will repeatedly encounter face validity and some of its consequences in subsequent chapters.

NOTES

1. The characteristics that we will be considering here are modified from those previously advanced by Kornetsky (1977) and by Mathysse and Haber (1975).

2. It may be that a particular model will apply to only a restricted range of clinical phenomena. As we shall see in Chapter 12, for example, the model developed there does not apply to all instances of anxiety reduction, broadly conceived. Thus, in evaluating a model, it is important to recognize that the model may be pertinent to a restricted clinical drug response. That does not mean, however, that the model is of no value; it does mean that it is of limited value.

3. A given value of r can be statistically different from zero even though its absolute value is low because, as the number of paired values increases, the value of r that is "statistically significant" can decrease to low values. On the other hand, the absolute value alone determines the predictive power inherent in the relationship of two variables. Thus, a low r value may be "significant" yet indicate that one variable can be only poorly predicted from another.

4. Strictly speaking, computation of IFE should incorporate a correction for the number of pairs involved in the determination of r. For our purposes, this correction can be ignored.

Section 5
Models of Clinical Drug Response

THE TRADITIONAL LINKAGE of pharmacology to medicine, and of behavioral pharmacology to psychiatry, has generated a research emphasis that is focused on a restricted group of drugs. These drugs can be classified in terms of their demonstrable clinical efficacy; the classes are the anxiolytics, the neuroleptics, the antidepressants, and lithium.

This mode of classification presents a problem. As we have seen, we will need to develop laboratory models of the different clinical responses that underlie the classifications themselves. We have also seen that we can apply a set of rules to guide us in such model building (Chapter 11). The question, then, is how well we can do in developing satisfactory models. We will examine this question in Chapters 12, 13, and 14.

As we do so, we should keep several points in mind. First, the classification upon which we are focusing excludes a number of drugs from consideration; the classification necessarily dictates an arbitrary selectivity. Second, the potential diversity of experimental outcome forces us to emphasize a relatively few behavioral procedures primarily applied to one species, the laboratory rat. Our task, after all, is not to itemize all behavioral effects of all drugs in all species but to examine a restricted range of laboratory phenomena in hopes of developing satisfactory models of clinical drug response.

The third point relates to the varying degrees of success achievable in developing such models. For the anxiolytics, we will be able to develop a reasonably satisfactory model, but we will have only limited success with the neuroleptics. The antidepressants and lithium will present a bleaker picture. No truly useful models for the antidepressants have yet been developed despite some promising beginnings; there are virtually no usable data pertinent to lithium.

However, despite only limited success in developing useful models of clinical drug response, we will get a better understanding of the process of model development. In addition, the process itself will provide us with a convenient way to organize a very large body of information.

Chapter 12
The Anxiolytics

IN THIS CHAPTER we will focus on a clinical drug response—behavioral change indicating a reduction in anxiety—due to one class of drugs—the anxiolytics. Our major purpose will be to develop a laboratory model of the clinical response to these drugs. First, however, let us briefly consider the clinical phenomenon upon which the clinical drug response is based.[1]

ANXIETY AND THE ANXIOLYTICS

Anxiety is a term that refers to the signs that may accompany anticipated danger, imaginary or real. The following are the major features of anxiety, as described in the *Diagnostic and Statistical Manual of Mental Disorders:* *

Although the specific manifestations of the anxiety vary from individual to individual, generally there are signs of motor tension, autonomic hyperactivity, apprehensive expectation, and vigilance and scanning.

(1) Motor tension. Shakiness, jitteriness, jumpiness, trembling, tension, muscle aches, fatigability, and inability to relax are common complaints. There may also be eyelid twitch, furrowed brow, strained face, fidgeting, restlessness, easy startle, and sighing respiration.

*Diagnostic and Statistical Manual of Mental Disorders, 3rd ed. Washington, D.C.: American Psychiatric Association, 1980.

(2) Autonomic hyperactivity. There may be sweating, heart pounding or racing, cold, clammy hands, dry mouth, dizziness, light-headedness, paresthesias (tingling in hands or feet), upset stomach, hot or cold spells, frequent urination, diarrhea, discomfort in the pit of the stomach, lump in the throat, flushing, pallor, and high resting pulse and respiration rate.

(3) Apprehensive expectation. The individual is generally apprehensive and continually feels anxious, worries, ruminates, and anticipates that something bad will happen to himself or herself (e.g., fear of fainting, losing control, dying) or to others (e.g., family members may become ill or injured in an accident).

(4) Vigilance and scanning. Apprehensive expectation may cause hyperattentiveness so that the individual feels "on edge," impatient, or irritable. There may be complaints of distractibility, difficulty in concentrating, insomnia, difficulty in falling asleep, interrupted sleep, and fatigue on awakening.

Note that these signs are necessarily based on verbal report.

The following two case histories will help to clarify the range of these symptoms:*

Case I: A 27-year-old, married electrician complains of dizziness, sweating palms, heart palpitations, and ringing of the ears of more than eighteen months' duration. He has also experienced dry throat, periods of uncontrollable shaking, and a constant "edgy" and watchful feeling that often interfered with his ability to concentrate. These feelings have been present most of the time over the previous two years; they have not been limited to discrete periods.

Because of these symptoms he had seen a family practitioner, a neurologist, a neurosurgeon, a chiropractor, and an ENT specialist. He had been placed on a hypoglycemic diet, received physiotherapy for a pinched nerve, and told he might have "an inner ear problem."

For the past two years he has had few social contacts because of his nervous symptoms. Although he has sometimes had to leave work when the symptoms became intolerable, he continues to work for the same company for which he has worked since his apprenticeship following high school graduation. He tends to hide his symptoms from his wife and children, to whom he wants to appear "perfect," and reports few problems with them as a result of his nervousness.

Case II: A 12-year-old, pubertal girl came for a consultation because of a one-year history of "nervousness." About a year before the consultation, her parents had separated. Their marriage had been apparently stable and outwardly satisfactory up until that time, and their child-rearing practices were unremarkable. Following her parents' separation, the patient developed several fears and a relatively persistent state of anxiety. She began to bite

*Spitzer, R.L., Skodol, A.E., Gibbon, M., and Williams, J.B.: *DSM III Case Book*. Washington, D.C.: American Psychiatric Association, 1981.

her nails and worry about the excellence of her school performance; she became afraid of the dark and appeared to live in a relatively constant state of apprehension. Her worries were mostly realistic, but greatly exaggerated. She was concerned about her appearance, felt awkward, and her shyness in social situations became more pronounced. She reported relatively constant feelings of nervousness and anxiety, which seemed to be exacerbated by almost any event in her life. She experienced no panic attacks and no specific fears upon separation from her parents, although she was occasionally worried about their safety without good reason.

The patient is a shy girl who often has difficulty making friends though she has developed lasting and close relationships with several peers. Her school performance has ranged from adequate to outstanding and has not declined in the past year.

During the interview her palms were sweating, it was hard for her to look at the examiner, and she was rather inhibited and tense. She denied persistent feelings of sadness and lack of interest in her environment, and she said she was able to enjoy things except for the times when her anxiety peaked. When questioned about guilt, she reported with difficulty that sometimes she felt that somehow she was responsible for her parents' separation or divorce although she really couldn't say how. Physical examination findings were unremarkable. Specifically, she had no goiter or exophthalmos, and thyroid indices were within normal limits. Neurologic findings were unremarkable except for a mild tremor of extended hands during the examination, but this did not interfere with fine-motor skills.

ANXIOLYTIC DRUGS

When patients suffering from the kinds of symptoms described above are given certain drugs, they report clear reduction in anxiety; these drugs are the *anxiolytics,* a class of drugs defined in terms of the clinical drug response that they produce. The three general groups of anxiolytics in general use are itemized in Table 12–1; selected representatives of each group are also provided.

There are three other types of drugs that are also used in the manage-

Table 12–1

A. Barbiturates	Amobarbital
	Phenobarbital
B. Propanediols	Meprobamate
	Tybamate
C. Benzodiazepines	Chlordiazepoxide
	Diazepam
	Oxazepam
	Chlorazepate
	Nitrazepam
	Lorazepam

ment of anxiety. One of these is the *antihistamines;* of this group, hydroxyzine and diphenhydramine are most often prescribed. There is, however, no clear evidence that the antihistamines specifically reduce anxiety in any way comparable to the drugs listed in Table 12–1. That is, the antihistamines, despite occasional practice, are not true anxiolytics.

A second type is the *antidepressants* (discussed in Chapter 14). In the context of anxiety, it is noteworthy that some patients who respond poorly to the anxiolytics listed in Table 12–1 do often respond well to antidepressants. These patients are those in whom anxiety is manifested as intense, situation-specific phobic reactions and panic attacks. This instance of drug response thus refines the clinical phenomenon to which the usual definition of anxiolytic applies (see Chapter 11, Note 2).

Finally we must consider *propranolol,* a drug that is unquestionably useful in the management of certain cardiovascular disorders. It is also a drug for which claims of anxiolytic activity have been made. Although propranolol may control anxiety in selected patients, there are now no compelling data indicating that this is a general phenomenon comparable to that characteristic of the drugs in Table 12–1 (see Altesman, Cole, and Weingarten, 1980). For this reason, propranolol is not generally recommended for clinical use; it is, nonetheless, relevant to the business of model construction, as we shall see later.

SECONDARY EFFECTS OF THE ANXIOLYTICS

The anxiolytics, like any other group of drugs, have a broad spectrum of effects; they are not exclusively anxiolytic. These secondary effects include (1) muscle relaxant, (2) anticonvulsant, and (3) sedative effects. The anxiolytics thus can reduce clinically observed muscle spasms and are also useful in the management of certain clinical disorders that result in convulsions. Their sedative effects are clinically useful as well. Sedation is characterized by reduction in movement, tendency to sleep ("drowsiness"), and minor motor incoordination. Among the anxiolytics, the barbiturates and propanediols are relatively more sedating than are the benzodiazepines. This differential can be summarized by a ratio that is analogous to the therapeutic ratio we considered in Chapter 3. That is, if we obtain an anxiolytic dose, AD, and a sedative dose, SD, then the ratio AD/SD incorporates dose–response information and reflects anxiolytic activity relative to sedative activity. For example, the AD/SD ratios for the benzodiazepines are consistently lower than are those for the barbiturates and the propanediols.

LIMITATIONS ON THE ANXIOLYTIC RESPONSE

As noted in Chapter 10, the clinical drug responses that we are considering are inherently behavioral in nature. That is, they take the form of verbal behavior (reports about symptoms) or abnormalities in motor behavior. We do, nonetheless, tend to think of phenomena such as anxiety as being not merely behavioral but *internal* states or feelings as well.

Despite this pervasive tendency, the fact of the matter is that the data themselves are behavioral—states or feelings can never be measured directly. This is not to say that such feelings and states do not exist; it is to say that behavior constitutes the only phenomenon used to measure drug effect. This fact presents some special problems.

These problems inhere in the fact that the reported verbal behavior is based on observation—either observation by others of the patient or self-observation by the patient. In the first case, the limitations involved, discussed in Chapter 2, are obvious; the basic problem is one of reliability. The same sorts of limitations apply when the observer is also the patient.

When people observe their own feelings, they tend to believe that they are especially good reporters. Perhaps this is so because the states reported have an intimacy that external events do not have—a headache is certainly more personal than a loud noise. Although such states are indeed more intimate, it does not follow that people are especially skilled at reporting their feelings. The certainty with which the presence of such feelings is perceived does not necessarily mean that attempts to communicate these feelings are equally certain.

Because reports of feelings involve language, another limitation must be added to those characteristic of any kind of observation. Language is imprecise in differentiating among feelings; people cannot distinguish among worry–anxiety–apprehension or diffidence–shyness–embarrassment nearly as reliably as they can among red–green–blue or sweet–sour–bitter (see Skinner, 1975). It may be this limitation that leads to the pervasive complaints about failures to communicate, to form "meaningful relationships." Be that as it may, observational data are of limited reliability. This means, in turn, that the precise documentation of a specific instance of anxiety reduction is relatively hard to come by. Furthermore, the determination of the optimal dose of anxiolytic for any one patient will necessarily be a rather unreliable affair. Thus, analysis of anxiolytic effects has relied on global phenomena based on large numbers of patients.[2]

Such analytic studies have led to two conclusions. First, there is no doubt that certain drugs do reduce anxiety, broadly defined; more particularly, they produce verbal reports of reduced anxiety, the only empirical basis upon which analysis can proceed. Second, just as evidence of symptom management must be taken at a general level, so too must information concerning the effective clinical doses of different drugs. They are, at best, "ball park" figures for the anxiolytics as well as for the other classes of drugs to be discussed in subsequent chapters.

A MODEL OF THE CLINICAL ANXIOLYTIC RESPONSE

Until about 25 years ago, the major anxiolytic drug was a barbiturate, phenobarbital. Toward the end of the 1950s, however, a second drug, meprobamate, began to be more widely used; shortly thereafter another, chlordiazepoxide, was also introduced. At the same time, Geller and Seifter (1960) introduced a procedure that came to form the basis for all other techniques used to detect the action of anxiolytic drugs.

The basic procedure described by Geller and Seifter involves a multiple schedule that also includes a punishment component. In one segment of the schedule (signaled by a tone, say), responding is reinforced at irregular intervals (i.e., the schedule is VI). In a second segment (signaled by a different stimulus), every response is reinforced (the schedule is FR1); however, these responses, each reinforced, are also each punished by the delivery of a brief, inescapable electric shock. The consequence of this arrangement is that, with training, stable levels of responding occur during the VI component, whereas very low levels ("suppressed" responding) occur during the FR1–punishment component.[3]

Geller and Seifter discovered that meprobamate and the barbiturates increased the levels of responding in the punishment component (see Table 10–3). In contrast, amphetamine and one neuroleptic (promazine; see Chapter 13) did not have this action. Two years later, Geller, Kulak, and Seifter (1962) reported that chlordiazepoxide shares the antipunishment effect of meprobamate and the barbiturates.

These findings can obviously form a basis for the construction of a laboratory model. The question is whether these behavioral changes due to anxiolytics meet the various criteria discussed in Chapter 11.

EVALUATING THE MODEL

CRITERION A: DIFFERENTIATION, FALSE POSITIVES, AND FALSE NEGATIVES

A number of procedures based on the basic Geller–Seifter technique have been used to study the anxiolytics. We will, however, emphasize only one of these because it has been by far the most extensively used to generate the kinds of systematic data needed in evaluating a model. Although it is certainly true that the general rules that have emerged from this procedure are also characteristic of other techniques, it is important to recognize that a few specific exceptions to these generalizations have been obtained with variations in procedure. These exceptions are, however, generally small in magnitude, occur over a restricted dose range, or have not been notably replicable (see Sepinwall and Cook, 1978). More to the point, such exceptions are to be expected; in fact, as we have already noted, it is because the particulars of technique can so powerfully determine behavioral outcome that it is necessary to focus on a restricted mode of measurement.

The technique we will consider in detail is the one that has been extensively evaluated by Cook and his coworkers. The procedure involves food-deprived rats that have been trained to lever-press on a multiple schedule that incorporates two components. In one component, characterized by steady illumination in the response chambers, food reinforcements are available on a VI30 schedule; in the second component, characterized by interrupted illumination, reinforcements are available on a FR schedule. Once performance has stabilized on this schedule, brief, inescapable electric shocks are added to the FR component. Thus, following this change, the animal can claim reinforcements at intervals that average 30 seconds in the first component; reinforcements plus punishment (shock) occur with every tenth response in the second component. A sample set of cumulative records obtained by Cook and Davidson (1973) with this punishment technique are shown in Figure 12–1.

The record at the left of the figure indicates that stable rates of responding are characteristic of both components before the introduction of shock; F indicates food-only periods (both components in this case); the dashed lines denoted as (P) indicate to-be-punished periods. The middle panel of Figure 12–1 shows that the stable rates characteristic of the VI component are maintained (the initial period indicated by F), whereas very low levels of responding are characteristic of the punishment component (food plus shock, $F + S$).

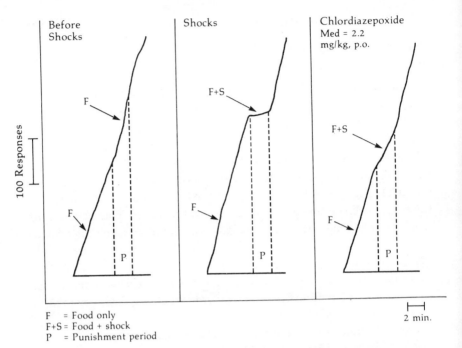

F   = Food only
F+S = Food + shock
P   = Punishment period

Figure 12–1. Cumulative records of responding maintained by a multiple schedule involving punishment; see text for details. (Redrawn from Cook and Davidson, 1973.)

The typical effect of the anxiolytic chlordiazepoxide is shown in the right-hand panel. Responding in the VI component (the initial period indicated by *F*) is essentially unaffected by drug, whereas behavior in the punishment component is dramatically different. In particular, the animal now responds (and sustains shock) at a substantial rate during a period in which essentially no responding occurred when drug was not given (the middle panel).

Cook and Davidson also studied a group of animals given different doses of chlordiazepoxide. The dose–response functions are shown in Figure 12–2; doses are plotted on logarithmic coordinates. The values shown are ratios of drug response to control response plotted on logarithmic coordinates; values greater than 1.0 (the horizontal line) thus indicate an increase in responding, and values less than 1.0, a decrease.

The solid curve in Figure 12–2 is the dose–response function obtained for responding in the punishment (FR) component; the dashed curve denotes the corresponding values for the unpunished (VI) component. Clearly, chlordiazepoxide produces a dose-dependent increase in re-

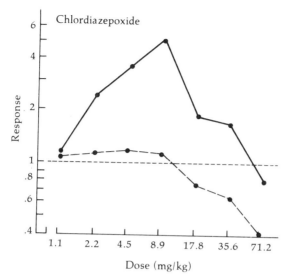

Figure 12–2. Dose–response function describing the effects of chlordiazepoxide on punished (solid line) and unpunished (dashed line) responding. (From Cook and Davidson, 1973.)

sponding to about 9.0 mg/kg; unpunished responding is unchanged over this dose range. At higher doses, responding declines. These decrements undoubtedly reflect the sedative property of chlordiazepoxide.

The differential effects of chlordiazepoxide on unpunished versus punished responding are reflected in the separation of the two dose–response functions in Figure 12–2. Compare this differential with the effects of the neuroleptic chlorpromazine, shown in Figure 12–3; for this agent, there is neither an overall increase in punished responding nor a marked separation of dose–response functions.

Comparison of the data in Figure 12–3 with those in Figure 12–2 will generate a variety of rules that differentiate chlordiazepoxide from chlorpromazine; the single rule adopted by Cook and Davidson is that, if a drug is to be classed as effective, it must produce a reliable increase in punished responding following drug at least two dose levels. Obviously, chlordiazepoxide is effective and chlorpromazine is ineffective.

Cook and Davidson (1973) used this criterion to assess the effects of a large number of drugs, each evaluated in a wide range of doses. The results of these assessments are summarized in Tables 12–2 and 12–3. Of the seven drugs that are clearly anxiolytic in clinical use (Groups A through C), all are effective in the laboratory model (see Table 12–1).

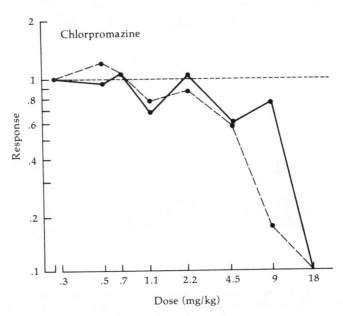

Figure 12–3. Dose–response function describing the effect of chlorpromazine on punished (solid line) and unpunished (dashed line) responding. (From Cook and Davidson, 1973.)

There are, however, three drugs (Group D) that are effective but are not clearly anxiolytic in clinical use.[4] Do these three entries qualify as false positives?

The problem inherent in answering this question is that the relevant clinical data are often not definitive. Lack of clearly demonstrable clinical activity of a drug obviously does not mean that it is devoid of that activity; this lack may mean only that it has not been properly evaluated. (A drug may not be systematically evaluated because its side-effects preclude clinical use. Thus, phencyclidine, for example, could be an anxiolytic but never have been carefully evaluated for that activity because it can also produce hallucinations.)

Therefore, we may sometimes be locked into a degree of uncertainty concerning false positives. For the moment, then, we must settle for the judgment that the model does generate false positives, even if that judgment is necessarily tentative.[5]

Although there is some ambiguity about all three entries in Group D, there is certainly no ambiguity about the single entry in Group E. There is no evidence that this neuroleptic is clinically anxiolytic, yet it is clearly effective in the model. It is, in fact, the most potent of the drugs listed.

Table 12–2
Effective Drugs

Group	Drug	MED (mg/kg, p.o.)
A. Barbiturates	Amobarbital	5.00
	Phenobarbital	4.50
B. Propanediols	Meprobamate	80.00
	Tybamate	62.50
C. Benzodiazepines	Chlordiazepoxide	2.20
	Diazepam	0.62
	Oxazepam	1.25
D. Other sedative hypnotics	Methaqualone	10.00
	Phencyclidine	4.40
	Benactyzine	4.50
E. Neuroleptics	Trifluoperazine	0.16

From Cook and Davidson, 1973.

Table 12–3
Ineffective Drugs

Group	Drugs	Dose tested (mg/kg) range
A. Neuroleptics	Haloperidol	0.03 – 0.48
	Chlorpromazine	0.27 – 17.90
B. Antidepressants	Iproniazid	20.00 –120.00
	Imipramine	0.55 – 17.70
C. Analgesics	Morphine	0.24 – 7.50
D. Antihistamines	Diphenhydramine	0.55 – 17.50
E. Sympathomimetics	Amphetamine	0.18 – 1.50
F. Antiadrenergics	Propranolol	2.5 – 80.0

From Cook and Davidson, 1973.

What is especially perplexing about this result is the fact that other neuroleptics (Group A in Table 12–3) are clearly ineffective. (This lack of effect of neuroleptics is also characteristic of results obtained in a very wide range of other punishment procedures; see Houser, 1978.) This result is, then, a conspicuous exception that may either be an important fact for future analysis or a laboratory curiosity.[6]

Let us now turn to Table 12–3 and reconsider several aspects of the discussion with which this chapter began. Recall that, despite some claims to the contrary, the antihistamines and propranolol have not been found to be consistently anxiolytic. These clinical findings agree with those presented in the table. Similar considerations apply to the antidepressants if we restrict our definition of clinical anxiety in such a way that it excludes phobic–panic reactions. We will have more to say about morphine and amphetamine later; for the moment we need note only that our model appears to be devoid of false negatives. That is, drugs lacking in clearly demonstrable clinical activity are ineffective in the model.

All in all, then, the model provides us with an impressive differentiation of anxiolytic from nonanxiolytic drugs. There are, to be sure, some ambiguous false positives (Group D in Table 12–1), one clear false positive (trifluoperazine), but no false negatives. Clearly, there must be factors controlling behavior in the model that are common to the behaviors that constitute the basis of our classification of drugs as anxiolytic.

CRITERION B: POTENCY RELATIONS

If there are indeed factors common to the two behaviors we are considering, then the clinical potencies of different known anxiolytics should correlate with their potencies in the model. The relevant data are given in Table 12–4. The parenthetical entries give the rank order of potencies within each set. The drugs have been arranged in order of decreasing clinical potency; diazepam is the most potent, meprobamate the least. The corresponding potencies based on the model show the same ordering with one exception—oxazepam is somewhat more potent than chlordiazepoxide in the model but not in the clinic. Obviously, then, the model is telling us something significant about clinical potency.

The correlation coefficient calculated from the seven pairs of values in Table 12–4 is equal to 0.997; the IFE is 92.2%. The relationship of

Table 12–4

Drug	Clinical Dose* (mg)		MED** (mg/kg)	
Diazepam	20	(1)	0.62	(1)
Chlordiazepoxide	40	(2)	2.20	(3)
Oxazepam	49	(3)	1.25	(2)
Phenobarbital	115	(4)	4.50	(4)
Amobarbital	175	(5)	5.00	(5)
Tybamate	1212	(6)	62.50	(6)
Meprobamate	1410	(7)	80.00	(7)

*Average daily oral doses, from Cook and Davidson (1973), except for tybamate, from Shader (1975).
**Data from Cook and Davidson, 1973.

clinical and laboratory potencies is shown in Figure 12–4. (This relationship can be more clearly visualized by using logarithmic coordinates.)
In short, in terms of Criterion B, the model is unquestionably a powerful
one.

CRITERION C: TEMPORAL CHARACTERISTICS

As we noted in Chapter 11, there are two temporal characteristics to
be considered: time of onset and tolerance. For the first characteristic,
clinical and laboratory phenomena show a good correspondence in that
the onset of pharmacologic activity is measured in minutes in both
cases. The second factor, tolerance, is somewhat more complex.

Although there is controversy about whether tolerance to anxiety reduction occurs as a consequence of chronic treatment with the benzodiazepines, there is little question that the sedative effects of these
drugs do show tolerance. This differential tolerance is paralleled in the

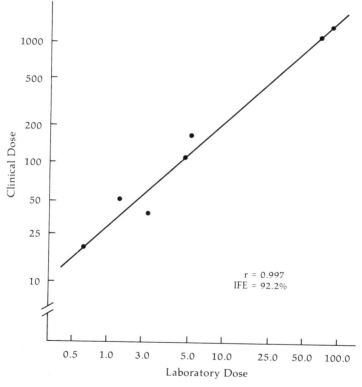

Figure 12–4. Relationship of laboratory dose to clinical dose for seven different anxiolytics (see Table 12–4).

model we are considering. The relevant data are shown in Figure 12–5.

In a study by Cook and Sepinwall (1975), animals that had been trained in the usual way were given a series of six weekly sessions; before each of these sessions they were given either a control dose of water (sessions *1* and *2*) or chlordiazepoxide (sessions *3* through *6*). The data are expressed, as usual, as ratios of post-drug responding to undrugged control responding (the "drug" was water in sessions *1* and *2*). Thus, values near 1.0 (the horizontal line) indicate no effect.

The dose of chlordiazepoxide is a high one (10.0 mg/kg; see Table 12–2), intentionally chosen to reduce the unpunished responding obtained in the VI component. This dose clearly had such an effect on unpunished responding in session *3*, at which time punished responding (in FR) was increased. More to the point, the sedative effect of the drug (indicated by the decrease in unpunished responding) clearly tolerates in the course of sessions *4* through *6*, whereas the antipunishment effect (indicative of anxiolytic activity) is clearly enhanced. Furthermore, this correspondence to the differential tolerance seen clinically is not restricted to this particular procedure (see Sepinwall and Cook, 1978; Sansone, 1979).

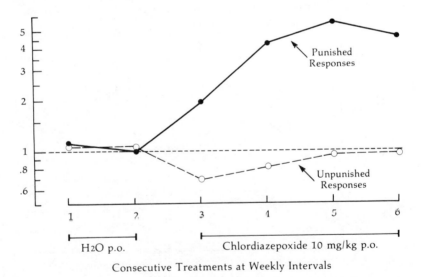

Figure 12–5. Differential tolerance of the changes in unpunished responding (an index of sedation) and punished responding (an index of anxiolysis); the former is characterized by tolerance, whereas the latter is not. (From Cook and Sepinwall, 1975.)

These facts suggest that the false positives previously discussed (Group D in Table 12–2) might be separated from the benzodiazepines on the basis of differential tolerance. That is, the Group D entries, all of which are quite sedating, may be characterized by a tolerance of their anxiolytic properties, whereas the benzodiazepines are not. Only studies of the effects of chronic administration of Group D drugs can answer this question.

Related questions pertain to the barbiturates. These anxiolytics are relatively more sedating than the benzodiazepines and are apparently characterized by tolerance of both their anxiolytic and sedating properties. We can thus ask: Would the model show a parallelism to these clinical phenomena? Again, only studies involving chronic treatment can answer the question.

Although these questions cannot now be answered, we can at least say that, for the benzodiazepines, the differential tolerance found in the clinic is mirrored in the model. Furthermore, there is a good correspondence of time to onset of pharmacologic activity in the clinic with that in the laboratory.

CRITERION D: DRUG INTERACTIONS

The most common drug interaction relevant to the clinical use of the anxiolytics is that with alcohol (ethanol). The anxiolytics can profoundly potentiate the actions of alcohol in humans.

Ethanol does have specific activity (the MED is 1000.00 mg/kg); it thus has a very low potency relative to the other drugs in Table 12–2. Although the clinical potentiation would be expected to be obtained in the model, this prospect has not been systematically evaluated.

CRITERION E: EVALUATIONS IN HUMANS

When we consider the relation of clinical and laboratory drug responses, we are immediately confronted by an analytic discrepancy: verbal report is not behavioral suppression, and rats cannot describe the effects the anxiolytics have on them. It is possible, however, to ask whether humans will suppress their behavior when confronted by punishment contingencies. Can we change species and obtain comparable behavioral effects? Unhappily, there are few answers to this question.

There are data suggesting that the behavioral effects of several drugs on humans are comparable to those seen in laboratory animals when humans are subjected to contingencies analogous to those used in the laboratory (Fischman, Schuster, and Uhlenhuth, 1977). The procedures used in these experiments are not, however, directly pertinent to our model. More directly comparable effects have been reported by Vogel-Sprott (1967).

In this study, human subjects were exposed to a procedure in which they were reinforced (by money) but were also punished (by electric shock). Vogel-Sprott found that, first, alcohol increased responding despite punishment and, second, this effect was relatively specific to the punishment situation (i.e., was attributable to neither a nonspecific tendency to respond nor to a measurable deficit in problem-solving). The essential features of this finding have been extended to the drug diazepam by Beer and Migler (1975).

In yet another experiment (Carlton, Siegel, Murphree, and Cook, 1981), ongoing responding (maintained by monetary reinforcement) was suppressed by punishment (monetary loss). (The subjects were, in effect, "gambling" in that running the risk of loss could also produce gain.) Diazepam was also found to antagonize punishment-induced suppression in this situation.

All three of these studies agree in indicating that effects comparable to those obtained in laboratory animals can also be obtained in humans. But this conclusion must be a very tentative one; it is derived, after all, from results of only three studies involving two anxiolytics (alcohol and diazepam) studied in single doses. There is no information about other anxiolytics, about nonanxiolytics, or about potency relations, temporal factors, or drug interactions. At the very best, we can say only that these data do not contradict what we would expect on the basis of our laboratory data.

This necessarily tentative conclusion about extensions to humans poses a very serious problem. In the first place, a complete analysis of pharmacologic effect will ultimately require a study of the drug in humans. Although not all of the experiments that are possible in the laboratory can be undertaken, at least some of the criteria in our earlier discussions should be plausibly met. Suitable analytic procedures are therefore required.

Unfortunately, the development of such techniques has generally been conspicuously unsuccessful (see Debus and Janke, 1980), perhaps because such development has relied almost exclusively on face validity, on procedures that look like they "should" induce anxiety. It is reasonable to suppose, on the other hand, that greater success will follow from procedures that mimic those that are demonstrably successful in laboratory animals and have already shown preliminary success in humans. It is certain that refined procedures applicable to humans will be needed ultimately, and it is likely that their development will proceed along lines already established in the laboratory.

NOTES

1. Individual studies relevant to the anxioloytics have been surveyed in valuable articles by Bignami (1978) and by Houser (1978).
2. That definitive data of this kind can be obtained is illustrated in the work of Rickels (e.g., Rickels, Downing, and Winokur, 1978).
3. These procedures are sometimes called "conflict" procedures because they seem to put the animal in a state of conflict about whether it should or should not respond. This label relies solely on face validity and implies a knowledge of the inner workings of the animal that is, in fact, not available. All in all, the usage is a bad idea.
4. Both methaqualone (Quaalude) and phencyclidine ("angel dust") are widely abused drugs. There is, however, no evidence that benactyzine and trifluoperazine (E in Table 12–2) are abused. Thus, anxiolytic activity itself is not a sure indicator of abuse potential.
5. Geller and Seifter (1962) have also reported that a group of drugs called *urethanes* antagonize punishment-induced suppression. There are no clinical data on these drugs so that it cannot be determined whether they are false or true positives. It is also noteworthy that anticholinergics such as atropine and scopolamine antagonize suppression induced in a variety of situations (see Bignami and Michalek, 1978). They do not, however, consistently antagonize punishment-induced suppression in situations of the kind considered here. Furthermore, there are no clear clinical indications that these anticholinergics are truly anxiolytic. They can thus be classed as true negatives.
6. Ethyl alcohol has also been found to antagonize suppression in situations closely allied to those discussed here.

Chapter 13
The Neuroleptics

LET US NOW extend our analysis of clinical drug response to a second class of drugs, the *neuroleptics,* used in the treatment of schizophrenia. This class, like the anxiolytics, is defined in terms of a particular drug response. We will focus, not on drug-induced changes in anxiety, but on drug-induced changes in schizophrenic behavior.[1]

SCHIZOPHRENIA AND THE NEUROLEPTICS

The neuroleptics are those drugs that have been found to be especially successful in the management of schizophrenic symptoms. We can get some idea of the magnitude of this success by considering Figure 13–1. As the figure implies, the introduction of the neuroleptics in 1956 produced, for the very first time, a reversal in an otherwise ever-increasing population of hospitalized patients. (The population has continued to decline since 1967 to a level of about 170,000.)

It is fair to say that no single event has had a greater impact on the care of schizophrenic patients than the introduction of the neuroleptics into psychiatric practice. Indeed, the neuroleptics, because they do so successfully control symptoms, made it possible to manage patients on a much more humane outpatient basis; the predominantly custodial "snake pit" became a thing of the past.[2] What, then, is the clinical phenomenon—schizophrenia—for which there is such a dramatic clinical drug response?

Number of Resident Patients in State and Local
Government Mental Hospitals in the United States
1946-1967

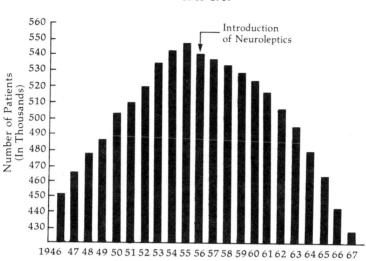

Figure 13–1. Number of hospitalized patients (in thousands) for the period 1946–1967. (Modified from Davis and Cole, 1975.)

The behavioral signs that contribute to the diagnosis of schizophrenia are varied and diffuse; a truly adequate description of the disorder would take us far afield. Let us focus on a few of the pivotal signs to get a general sense of the phenomenon. A patient may be considered schizophrenic if at least one of the following symptoms emerges during a phase of the illness:*

1. Bizarre delusions (content is patently absurd and has no possible basis in fact)
2. Somatic, grandiose, religious, nihilistic, or other delusions
3. Delusions of persecutory or jealous content if accompanied by hallucinations of any type
4. Auditory hallucinations in which either a voice keeps up a running commentary on the individual's behavior or thoughts, or two or more voices converse with each other
5. Auditory hallucinations on several occasions with content of more

*Criteria modified from *Diagnostic and Statistical Manual of Mental Disorders,* 3rd ed. Washington, D.C.: American Psychiatric Association, 1980.

than one or two words, having no apparent relation to depression or elation

6. Incoherence, marked loosening of associations, markedly illogical thinking, or marked poverty of content of speech if associated with at least one of the following:

(a) blunted, flat, or inappropriate affect

(b) delusions or hallucinations

(c) catatonic or other grossly disorganized behavior

In addition, the patient shows a clear deterioration of functioning in such areas as work, self-care, and social relations. Finally, continuous signs of schizophrenia must have been present for at least six months at some point in the patient's life and some signs must be currently present.

The following transcript of a case presentation gives some idea of the range of these symptoms:*

You have before you today a strongly built and well-nourished man, aged twenty-one, who entered the hospital a few weeks ago. He sits quietly looking in front of him, and does not raise his eyes when he is spoken to, but evidently understands all our questions very well, for he answers quite relevantly, though slowly and often only after repeated questioning. From his brief remarks, made in a low tone, we gather that he thinks he is ill, without getting any more precise information about the nature of the illness and its symptoms. The patient attributes his malady to the onanism (masturbation) he has practised since he was ten years old. He thinks that he has thus incurred the guilt of a sin against the sixth commandment, has very much reduced his power of working, has made himself feel languid and miserable, and has become a hypochondriac. Thus, as the result of reading certain books, he imagined that he had a rupture and suffered from wasting of the spinal cord, neither of which was the case. He would not associate with his comrades any longer, because he thought they saw the results of his vice and made fun of him. The patient makes all these statements in an indifferent tone, without looking up or troubling about his surroundings. His expression betrays no emotion; he only laughs for a moment now and then. There is occasional wrinkling of the forehead or facial spasm. Round the mouth and nose a fine, changing twitching is constantly observed.

The patient gives us a correct account of his past experiences. His knowledge speaks for the high degree of education; indeed, he was ready to enter the University a year ago. He also knows where he is and how long he has been here, but he is only very imperfectly acquainted with the

---

*Spitzer, R.L., Skodol, A.E., Gibbon, M., and Williams, J.B.: *DSM III Case Book*. Washington, D.C.: American Psychiatric Association, 1981.

names of the people round him, and says that he has never asked about them. He can only give a very meagre account of the general events of the last year. In answer to our questions he declares that he is ready to remain in the hospital for the present. He would certainly prefer it if he could enter a profession, but he cannot say what he would like to take up . . . The patient makes his statements slowly and in monosyllables, not because his wish to answer meets with overpowering hindrances, but because he feels no desire to speak at all. He certainly hears and understands what is said to him very well, but he does not take the trouble to attend to it. He pays no heed, and answers whatever occurs to him without thinking. No visible effort of the will is to be noticed. All his movements are languid and expressionless, but are made without hindrance or trouble. There is no sign of emotional dejection, such as one would expect from the nature of his talk, and the patient remains quite dull throughout, experiencing neither fear nor hope nor desires. He is not at all deeply affected by what goes on before him, although he understands it without actual difficulty. It is all the same to him who appears or disappears, where he is or who talks to him and takes care of him, and he does not even once ask their names.

. . . He broods, staring in front of him with expressionless features, over which a vacant smile occasionally plays, or at the best turns over the leaves of a book for a moment, apparently speechless, and not troubling about anything. Even when he has visitors, he sits without showing any interest, does not ask about what is happening at home, hardly even greets his parents, and goes back indifferently to the ward. He can hardly be induced to write a letter, and says that he has nothing to write about. But he occasionally composes a letter to the doctor, expressing all kinds of distorted, half-formed ideas, with a peculiar and silly play on words, in very fair style, but with little connection. He begs for "a little more allegro in the treatment" and "liberationary movement with a view to the widening of the horizon" will "ergo extort some wit in lectures," and "nota bene for God's sake only does not wish to be combined with the club of the harmless." "Professional work is the balm of life."

The development of the illness has been quite gradual. Our patient . . . did not go to school till he was seven years old, as he was a delicate child and spoke badly, but when he did he learned quite well. He was considered to be a reserved and stubborn child. Having practised onanism at a very early age, he became more and more solitary in the last few years, and thought that he was laughed at by his brothers and sisters, and shut out from society because of his ugliness. For this reason, he could not bear a looking-glass in his room. After passing the written examination on leaving school, a year ago, he gave up the viva voce, because he could not work any longer. He cried a great deal, masturbated much, ran about aimlessly, played in a senseless way on the piano, and began to write observations " 'On the Nerve-play of Life' which he cannot get on with." He was incapable of any kind of work, even physical, felt "done for," asked for a revolver, ate Swedish matches to destroy himself, and lost all affection for his family. From time to time he became excited and troublesome, and shouted out the window at night. In the hospital, too, a state of excitement lasting for several days was observed, in which he chattered in a confused way, made faces, ran about at full speed, wrote disconnected scraps of composition, and crossed and recrossed them with flourishes and unmeaning combinations of letters. After this a state of tranquility ensued, in which he could give absolutely no account of his extraordinary behavior.

NEUROLEPTIC DRUGS

There are several classes of neuroleptics, as shown in Table 13–1. Representatives of each class and their approximate daily doses are also shown.

LIMITATIONS OF THE CLINICAL DRUG RESPONSE

The various behaviors that are characterized as schizophrenic are obviously either reports of the patients (of hallucinations, for example) or of others who report about the patient (of their bizarre actions, for example). Thus, the clinical response with which we are concerned (remission of these symptoms) is based on observational data in precisely the

Table 13–1

Neuroleptic Class	Drug	Median Daily Dose* (mg)
Phenothiazines	Promazine	2085
	Chlorpromazine	750
	Thioridazine	788
	Mesoridazine	412
	Prochlorperazine	105
	Triflupromazine	285
	Perphenazine	68
	Trifluoperazine	22
	Fluphenazine	8
Thioxanthenes	Chlorprothixene	330
	Thiothixene	38
Butyrophenones	Haloperidol	8
Indolones	Molindone	112
Dibenzazepines	Clozapine**	1538
Diphenylbutyl piperidines	Pimozide**	8

*Data derived from daily dose ranges in Creese, Burt, and Snyder (1976), Davis and Cole (1975), and, for molindone, Shader (1975).
**Experimental drugs

same way as were the data pertinent to the clinical anxiolytic response.
    In addition to the limitations that the nature of these reports imposes,
there is a second kind of limitation, which inheres in the fact that not
all symptoms are equally affected by the neuroleptics. As a rough rule,
the symptoms itemized in category A in Table 13–2 can definitely be
expected to be controlled by the neuroleptics, whereas those in categories B through D have varying degrees of likelihood of response.Note
that the table does not include a specific entry for anxiety. Although
schizophrenic patients may have anxiety symptoms, the neuroleptics
are not particularly effective in controlling this anxiety. Furthermore,
the neuroleptics are clearly not effective anxiolytics when given to non-
schizophrenic patients; conversely, the anxiolytics are of essentially no
value in controlling schizophrenic behaviors.[3]
    There is, thus, a specificity of clinical drug response—a specificity that
also extends to the antidepressants that we will consider in the next
chapter: the antidepressants are of no clear value in the management
of schizophrenia, and the neuroleptics are generally of little value in
controlling clinical depression.[4]

SECONDARY EFFECTS OF THE NEUROLEPTICS

Table 13–2 makes it clear that not all symptoms of schizophrenia are
equally well-controlled by the neuroleptics. Furthermore, the effects of
these drugs are not restricted to the target symptoms themselves. In fact,
the neuroleptics have a broad range of effects other than those directly
pertinent to schizophrenia.

Table 13–2*

Category	Symptoms	Likelihood of response
A.	Thinking disorder Withdrawal Hyperactivity Uncooperativeness Competitiveness	Definite
B.	Hallucinations Paranoid delusions Hostility	Probable
C.	Flat affect	Possible
D.	Disorientation Lack of insight	Minimal

*Adapted from Honigfeld and Howard, 1978.

The major secondary effects with which we will be concerned are the following:

1. Sedative
2. Antihistaminic: effects like those produced by antihistamines
3. Anticholinergic: effects comparable to those produced by atropine or scopolamine; see Chapter 3
4. Adrenergic blocking actions: see Chapter 17
5. Extrapyramidal symptoms (EPS): the array of motor symptoms that are collectively called EPS include transient loss of muscle tone (dystonic reactions), motor restlessness (akathisia), and a parkinsonian syndrome (including motor retardation, rigidity, and tremor)

Some of these secondary effects will be discussed in greater detail in later chapters.

A MODEL OF THE CLINICAL NEUROLEPTIC RESPONSE

Courvoisier first reported (1953) that the neuroleptic chlorpromazine produced a loss of avoidance responding maintained in animals previously trained in a discriminated avoidance procedure. This basic finding was later elaborated by Cook and Weidley (1957), Maffii (1959), Cook and Catania (1964), and Davidson and Weidley (1976), as well as by a number of others (see Bignami, 1978).

The characteristic sign of neuroleptic activity is, first, a differential loss of avoidance behavior with, second, relatively little loss in escape responding. Recall that, in discriminated avoidance, the animal has the opportunity to avoid impending electric shock by emitting a prescribed response to a warning signal. If the animal fails to emit the avoidance response, shock occurs; the animal can then escape the shock by emitting the prescribed response. The neuroleptics produce decrements in avoidance responding even though escape responding is maintained. A sample set of data, from a study by Cook and Sepinwall (1975), is shown in Figure 13–2. The figure indicates that increasing doses of chlorpromazine produce progressively greater deficits in avoidance (indicated as percent inhibition). Furthermore, these deficits can persist up to 24 to 28 hours after injection. (Note, especially, the 20-mg/kg dose at the bottom of the figure.) At no point is there a reliable deficit in escape responding. Thus, after 10 mg/kg, for example, previously trained rats that had never failed to avoid prior to drug administration (0% inhibition) show a peak of 80% loss two hours after drug. At no point do they fail to escape.

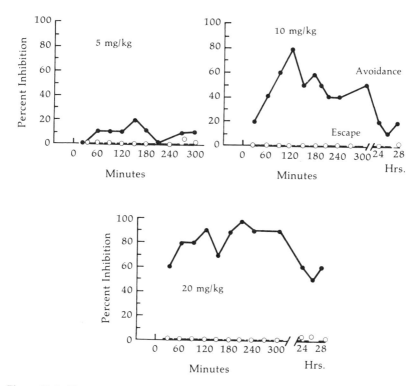

Figure 13–2. Time course of effect of different doses of chlorpromazine on avoidance and escape responding in a discriminated avoidance situation. (From Cook and Sepinwall, 1975.)

This differential effect is, of course, dose-dependent. At chlorpromazine doses higher than those shown in Figure 13–2, deficits in escape responding do occur; see Figure 13–3. In the study by Cook and Catania (1964), increasing doses of chlorpromazine produced a dose-dependent inhibition of avoidance responding in the range of 5.0–40.0 mg/kg. (The plotted values in Figure 13–3 are the maximum levels of inhibition obtained in the post-drug session.) In contrast, a reliable inhibition of escape behavior was obtained only at the 40.0 mg dose. Differential effects of this kind can be summarized in terms of a ratio of doses: the dose that produces a given level of avoidance loss—ED_{50}-AL—relative to the dose that produces the same level of escape loss—ED_{50}-EL. The ratios of these doses will be low to the extent that there is a selective effect on avoidance responding (i.e., avoidance loss, AL, occurs at doses less than those at which escape loss, EL, occur).

We have thus far considered only one neuroleptic—chlorpromazine. The question to which we now turn is whether discriminated avoidance

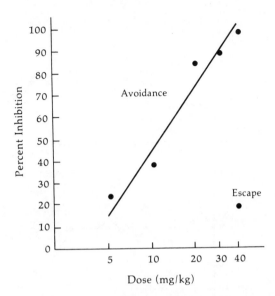

Figure 13–3. Dose–response function for the effects of chlorpromazine on discriminated avoidance responding; a relatively small inhibition of escape responding occurs only at the highest dose. (Adapted from Cook and Catania, 1964.)

will provide us with a satisfactory laboratory model. In answering this question, we will, as we did in the case of the anxiolytics, restrict ourselves to our prototype species, the laboratory rat. In addition, we will, as before, examine only a few procedures, those that provide data sufficiently systematic for our purposes. In particular, we will focus on the reports by Cook and Weidley (1957), Maffii (1959), Cook and Catania (1964), and Davidson and Weidley (1976); in addition, we will consider a largely neglected report by Pfeiffer and Jenney (1957). Although this emphasis is a restricted one, there is no question that the general results apply to a very broad range of discriminated avoidance procedures (see Bignami, 1978).

EVALUATING THE MODEL

CRITERION A: DIFFERENTIATION, FALSE POSITIVES, AND FALSE NEGATIVES

The first question that we must ask is whether discriminated avoidance differentiates neuroleptics from non-neuroleptics. As a first step in examining Criterion A, let us turn to the study by Cook and Weidley (1957).

In this study, chlorpromazine, reserpine, and morphine were all found to produce specific attenuation of avoidance (i.e., ED_{50}-AL clearly lower than ED_{50}-EL). The first two drugs are established neuroleptics, but morphine is not. In addition, Cook and Weidley found that meprobamate, pentobarbital, and barbital had nonspecific effects (i.e., their ED_{50}-ALs and ED_{50}-ELs were essentially identical).

Maffii (1959) replicated the data concerning chlorpromazine, reserpine, morphine, meprobamate, and several barbiturates. He also extended the analysis to another neuroleptic (promazine), an antidepressant (iproniazid), and a hallucinogen (mescaline). Promazine, like chlorpromazine, had a specific effect, but the other two drugs did not.

These data indicate that discriminated avoidance is selectively sensitive to the neuroleptics. There is, however, one false positive, morphine. Unfortunately, there are others.

Pfeiffer and Jenney (1957) studied the effects of several drugs, all cholinomimetics (see Chapter 3), and found that all produced specific effects on discriminated avoidance analogous to those produced by the neuroleptics. Table 13–3 summarizes all of the preceding data.Table 13–3 makes it clear that our model provides substantial differentiation among the three major drug classes we are considering. Neuroleptics uniformly have specific effects, whereas the anxiolytics and the antidepressants have nonspecific effects.

Although no false negatives have been reported, it is clear that the model is sensitive to drugs that may be false positives (morphine and the cholinomimetics). When we consider these drugs we are immediately confronted by the same problem we met in considering Criterion A in Chapter 12: Are these drugs truly false positives or have they merely been inadequately evaluated in the clinic?

As it happens, Pfeiffer and Jenney also reported that cholinomimetics given to schizophrenics could produce transient "lucid intervals" in these patients. Although there have been occasional confirmatory reports since that time, it is certainly true that the cholinomimetics are in no way clinically comparable to the neuroleptics in the symptom

Table 13–3

Specific Effects	Nonspecific Effects
Neuroleptics	Antidepressants
Morphine	Anxiolytics
Cholinomimetics	

management they provide. Thus, it appears that these drugs are truly false positives.

The other potential false positive is morphine, a drug that Cook and Weidley as well as Maffii reported to have specific effects. (Comparable results were also reported by Verhave, Owen, and Robbins, 1959). But does morphine have neuroleptic activity as defined in terms of clinical efficacy?

It may be, of course, that morphine has not been systematically evaluated because of its addiction liability. It is, nonetheless, reasonable to suppose that morphine has been used for the control of pain in patients who were also schizophrenic. Had a dramatic remission of schizophrenic symptoms consistently occurred, there would surely be a substantial literature documenting this fact—but there is not. Thus, morphine also appears to be a genuine false positive.[5]

Despite these false positives, our model does provide a reasonable degree of differentiation between neuroleptics and non-neuroleptics. This outcome naturally leads us to Criterion B: Do the laboratory potencies of different neuroleptics predict their clinical potencies?

CRITERION B: POTENCY RELATIONS

There are many neuroleptics available for clinical use, but as far as efficacy alone is concerned, no one drug is superior to any other. That is, no neuroleptic has been shown to be reliably superior to any other in terms of controlling schizophrenic behaviors. Although there is no "better" neuroleptic, however, different neuroleptics do vary widely in their potencies (i.e., in the amounts required to produce optimal symptom control). The average daily dose of chlorpromazine, for example, is about 750 mg, whereas the corresponding value for fluphenazine is about 8 mg, a 90-fold difference (see Table 13–1). The question we must now address is whether these potencies are correlated with those obtained in our model; let us focus on the report by Davidson and Weidley (1976) because it provides the largest amount of data.

Davidson and Weidley studied the effects of all 15 of the neuroleptics itemized in Table 13–1. The drugs were evaluated during the acquisition of discriminated avoidance responding; naive animals that had no previous training were injected and then given 100 avoidance trials.

The dose required to reduce levels of avoidance to 50% of control (i.e., ED_{50}-AL) for each neuroleptic is given in Table 13–4. The percent loss of escape responding for each drug at its ED_{50}-AL is also shown in the table. Promazine, for example, produced a 50% avoidance loss at 24.7 mg/kg but only a 5% deficit in escape responding (i.e., the difference at the ED_{50}-AL is thus 45%). Looked at in this way, the procedure clearly provides the characteristic difference in effects on avoidance versus escape behaviors.

Plotting these laboratory doses against the clinical doses given in Table 13–1 yields the relationship shown in Figure 13–4. The correlation coefficient of these values is 0.870, which generates an IFE of 50.7%. These values indicate that the acquisition of discriminated avoidance provides for less predictability of clinical dose than that possible with punishment procedures used with the anxiolytics (IFE = 92.2%; Figure 12–4). In terms of Criterion B, then, discriminated avoidance certainly does provide us with a useful model, although it is less powerful when compared with punishment procedures.[6]

CRITERION C: TEMPORAL CHARACTERISTICS

Our model does reasonably well in differentiating neuroleptics from non-neuroleptics (Criterion A) and predicts clinical potency (Criterion B). There are, however, several false positives, and the IFE is relatively low (50.7%). Our model is, in short, not without its problems, and more of them lie ahead.

One of these has to do with the time of onset of neuroleptic activity

Table 13–4

Drug	ED_{50}-AL (mg/kg)	Percentage Escape Loss
Promazine	24.70	5
Clozapine	7.20	0
Mesoridazine	6.50	2
Thioridazine	5.00	0
Molindone	2.50	2
Chlorprothixene	1.90	15
Thiothixene	1.90	7
Chlorpromazine	1.80	0
Triflupromazine	0.87	7
Prochlorperazine	0.44	1
Fluphenazine	0.37	20
Trifluoperazine	0.30	0
Perphenazine	0.24	11
Pimozide	0.23	0
Haloperidol	0.16	3

From Davidson and Weidley, 1976.

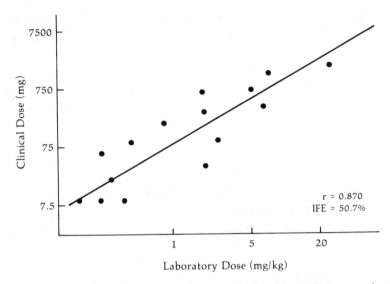

Figure 13–4. Relationship of laboratory dose to clinical dose for 15 different neuroleptics (see Tables 13–1 and 13–4).

in the clinic versus the laboratory. Neuroleptics do have rapid effects in humans; full remission of symptoms is, however, measured in days, not minutes. In contrast, effects on discriminated avoidance appear within minutes. There is, thus, a disparity between the onset of the clinical drug response and the laboratory response. This disparity leads directly to another consideration.

Although the clinical data are not as precise as we would want, it can be said that the onset of at least some signs of motor dysfunction (ESP) following initiation of neuroleptic treatment is, if anything, more rapid than the onset of symptom control. There is, therefore, a roughly closer temporal correspondence of EPS and avoidance loss than there is of symptom remission and avoidance loss.

This is not a definitive conclusion because the available data are not sufficiently precise. The suggestion does, nonetheless, sound a thematic note to which we will return again and again. Is our model more closely related to EPS than to clinical drug response? A part of the answer to this question is provided by considering the issue of tolerance.

We know that EPS may wane in the face of chronic neuroleptic medication, whereas symptom remission does not; there is a dissociation of EPS and clinical drug response. The question then becomes the following: do the effects of neuroleptics on discriminated avoidance show tolerance (parallel EPS) or fail to show tolerance (parallel clinical drug response)?

The data relevant to this question are also not as definitive as we would want. We can say only that there is no compelling evidence indicating that tolerance does characterize the effects of neuroleptics on discriminated avoidance. The data in Figure 13–5 are a case in point.

Laffan, High, and Burke (1965) studied the effects of daily injections of fluphenazine at two dose levels; the values in the left panel of Figure 13–5 have been estimated from the graphic presentation in their report. Clearly, there is a dose-dependent increase in avoidance loss; there is no evidence for a waning of effect in the course of the six days of the experiment. Comparable results have been reported by Kuribara and Tadokoro (1979); these are shown in the right panel of Figure 13–5. In this study, a long-acting form of fluphenazine was injected at weekly intervals. Again, there is a dose-dependent avoidance loss, with little evidence for tolerance.

This general conclusion is also supported by other studies reported both by Laffan, High, and Burke and by Kuribara and Tadokoro (also see the discussion by Clody and Beer, 1975). Despite the consensus

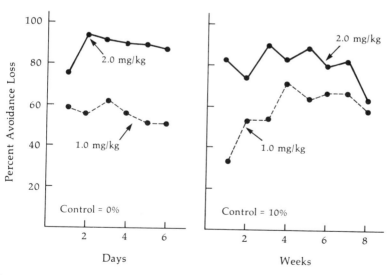

Figure 13–5. *Left,* Effects of two doses of fluphenazine given daily. *Right,* Effects of a long-acting form of fluphenazine given weekly. (Modified from Laffan, High and Burke, 1965, and from Kuribara and Tadokoro, 1979.)

about a lack of tolerance, this conclusion must be viewed with at least moderate caution, for several reasons:

In the first place, the studies have emphasized only one neuroleptic, fluphenazine. Therefore, whether a lack of tolerance is generally characteristic of all neuroleptics is an open question. A second reservation about these data has to do with the completeness of the reports from which they are taken. The key to differentiating the neuroleptics lies in their differential effects on avoidance versus escape responding. Unfortunately, the degree of separation of these two effects (e.g., ED_{50}-AL versus ED_{50}-EL) in the course of chronic treatment has not been systematically reported. Thus, we know that avoidance loss is maintained, but we cannot be certain that the unique sign of neuroleptic action (avoidance versus escape) is comparably maintained.

Finally, there is the problem of missing dose–response information. As we have repeatedly noted, the absence of such data in analyzing tolerance can lead to misguided conclusions (see Chapter 8). Accordingly, when we consider this prospect in combination with the previous three, we can conclude only that tolerance has not been compellingly demonstrated to be a characteristic effect of the neuroleptics on our laboratory model. We can also conclude that the question has not been scrutinized to the desired degree.[7]

CRITERION D: DRUG INTERACTIONS

The interaction that we will consider here has to do with a single group of drugs—the anticholinergics. These drugs antagonize the effects of the neuroleptics in our model (see Cook and Sepinwall, 1976). This fact is an important one because of the following:

1. Anti-EPS medications are generally anticholinergic.
2. They do antagonize EPS due to the neuroleptics.
3. They do *not* antagonize the clinical drug response (reduction in schizophrenic symptoms) due to neuroleptics.

It is, therefore, possible to dissociate the clinical drug response from our laboratory drug response on the basis of a selective antagonism. This conclusion brings us back to the suggestion that our model may be linked to EPS, rather than to the clinical drug response per se. We will consider this prospect in greater detail in Chapter 16.

CRITERION E: EVALUATIONS IN HUMANS

As noted in the last chapter, any adequate development of a model requires that the analysis be brought full circle, back to humans. We begin with a clinical phenomenon, link that phenomenon to a laboratory model via drug response, and, in the process, examine the validity of the model. But the circle will be completed only when the model is applied to humans in order to determine the extent to which the laboratory phenomena can be realized in this species. Clearly, if our model does not hold up when the species *is* human, it cannot be regarded as a satisfactory one. Unfortunately, there are only minimal data bearing on the issue.

One relevant study has been reported by Cook and Catania (1964), who examined the effects of a low, single dose of chlorpromazine (37.5 mg., i.m.) given to human volunteers. (This dose is roughly one-twentieth of the average daily therapeutic dose.) These subjects had been trained to avoid shock on a nondiscriminated avoidance schedule that included an escape contingency. That is, if the subject failed to avoid, brief shocks were administered until the subject depressed the response lever and thus escaped. Data for one subject are summarized in Table 13–5. Response rate prior to injection (Period 1) was 5.8 responses per minute, and no shocks were received; therefore, there was no opportunity for escape. Following drug (Periods 2 through 4), response rate progressively declined and then recovered. The course of the changes in response rate produced a complementary increase in shocks received. This increase in the number of shocks provided an opportunity for escape responding; the increase in numbers of escape responses per minute is shown in the fourth column of the table. This increase in escape responding generates a

Table 13–5*

Period	Responses/min	Shocks/min	Escapes/min	Escape failure
1	5.8	0	0	0
		-(Injection)-		
2	3.9	0.5	0.5	0
3	1.3	1.8	1.2	0.6
4	4.9	0.1	0.1	0

*Estimated values, grouped into arbitrary periods for purposes of simplicity in presentation; data from Cook and Catania (1964).

question. On how many occasions was there a *failure* to escape?

If the subject emitted an escape response following each shock, then escapes per minute would equal shocks per minute, and the difference would be zero. Failure to escape is therefore indicated by a positive difference between shocks per minute and escapes per minute. These indices of escape failure are shown in the last column of the table.

The data indicate that the effects of chlorpromazine seen in our model can also be obtained in humans. That is, avoidance responding is decreased, but escape responding is maintained. In particular, note that, during the peak effect in Period 3, escape failure is only one third (0.6) of the maximum possible (1.8). Also note that there are no escape failures during Periods 2 and 4; that is, shocks do occur, but all are escaped. Furthermore, there is an indication that this selective effect is not characteristic of meprobamate, chlordiazepoxide, or phenobarbital (see Cook and Sepinwall, 1975). Thus, the anxiolytics can evidently be differentiated from chlorpromazine, just as they can be in the rat.

These results have been extended by Fischman and Schuster (1979; also see Fischman, Smith, and Schuster, 1976). Of particular interest is their use of a "point loss" procedure analogous to the avoidance procedure described by Cook and Catania. With this technique, subjects begin the experimental session with a number of "points" that are redeemable for money at the end of the session. During the session, however, they can lose points if they fail to respond (these points are tabulated on a counter visible to the subjects). Subjects can thus avoid point loss (and subsequent monetary loss) by responding on a nondiscriminated avoidance schedule. If, however, an initial loss does occur, subsequent losses occur at a relatively rapid rate (analogous to the shock delivery schedule in the experiment of Cook and Catania). Subjects can escape from these periods by responding. The procedure thus provides for indices of avoidance responding, escape responding, and escape failure.

Fischman and her coworkers obtained dose-dependent decreases in avoidance responding due to both chlorpromazine and pentobarbital. More to the point, pentobarbital also produced an increase in escape failure, whereas chlorpromazine did not (see Table 13–5). The results are therefore congruent with those obtained by Cook and Catania.

Results of this kind are encouraging but certainly not definitive. The data parallel those obtained in our model, but they do not yet include sufficient dose–response information on a number of drugs (relevant to

Criteria A and B). Furthermore, interactions with the anticholinergics have not been examined, and there is no information on the effects of chronic medication.

These data are, however, encouraging on another score: They indicate that extensions of a laboratory procedure to humans will prove to be a useful undertaking. Such a statement cannot be made for most of the other techniques that have been used to explore the effects of the neuroleptics in humans.

Janke (1980) has provided us with an excellent review of the results obtained with the very broad range of procedures that have been used to study acute effects of neuroleptics administered to normal volunteers.[8] In general, these procedures have proved to be either insensitive to neuroleptic action or, if they are sensitive, unable to differentiate neuroleptics from other classes of drugs (Criterion A).

It therefore seems likely that useful procedures applicable to normal humans will be developed from those that are demonstrably useful in laboratory animals. It is certain that some such technique will be needed if the analysis of neuroleptic action is to be completed.

NOTES

1. The neuroleptics are effective in managing the symptoms of a broad range of psychotic disorders, of which schizophrenia is one. The major use of neuroleptics is, however, in treating schizophrenia; more to the point, the systematic data available pertain to this use.
2. Other factors (e.g., social attitudes about mental disease) undoubtedly contributed to this dramatic turnabout; it would be a mistake to say that the introduction of the neuroleptics was the only factor involved. This fact does not, however, reduce the significance of the neuroleptics in revolutionizing the care of schizophrenic patients.
3. There is a widely held belief that the neuroleptics are also anxiolytic. Thus, they have come to be called "tranquilizers." The usage is unfortunate because, although it is true that some neuroleptics may produce sedation, there are no systematic data indicating that they are truly anxiolytic.
4. One neuroleptic, thioridazine, appears to be an exception to this rule in that there is consistent evidence that it is effective in managing depression in at least some patients.
5. Morphine can, however, be differentiated from the neuroleptics on an experimental basis. In particular, Cook and Weidley found that

the opiate antagonist naloxone reversed the selective effect of morphine, but not of chlorpromazine, on discriminated avoidance.

6. Cook and Catania reported a parallel correlation based on seven neuroleptics. They reported an r of 0.913; IFE $= 59.3\%$ (median clinical values were used in the calculation).

7. The same animals were repeatedly tested in generating the data in Figure 13–5. This fact further complicates our interpretation of these data.

   Recall that Clody and Beer (Chapter 9 and Tables 9–4 and 9–5) found that repeated testing of the same animals produced a prolongation of the avoidance deficit; such a decrement in responding is, of course, the index of tolerance used in Figure 13–5. Thus, repeated testing could have increased the magnitude of deficit and could therefore have contributed to an apparent lack of tolerance (i.e., some tolerance might have been observed had different animals been used in single tests following different numbers of injections).

8. Mirsky and Kornetsky (1968) have reviewed important data indicating that the effects of neuroleptics can be differentiated from the effects of other drugs in schizophrenic patients rather than in normal subjects.

Chapter 14
Lithium and the Antidepressants

OUR MODEL OF clinical response for the anxiolytics (Chapter 12) is obviously well validated, whereas the model for the neuroleptics (Chapter 13) is somewhat weaker on several counts. The material covered in this chapter presents a picture that is bleaker still. In fact, as we shall see, there are no satisfactory models of the clinical response to either lithium or the antidepressants. Why, then, consider the data at all?

There are three general reasons: First, the data are of interest in their own right; second, they may ultimately generate useful models even though they have not yet done so. Third, the procedures discussed here provide an unusually clear instance of the kinds of problems that a reliance on face validity can produce. Before we address these concerns, however, we must consider the specific clinical phenomena relevant to lithium and the antidepressants: mania and depression, respectively. The prevalence of each disorder is substantial, and there are specific medications for each.

MANIA AND LITHIUM

Mania is a disorder characterized by hyperactivity, pressure of speech, grandiosity, flight of ideas, and belligerence, which may be seen intermittently and in varying degrees. Affected patients appear to be euphoric and have racing thoughts, delusions of grandeur, and poor if not self-destructive judgment. Manic patients are on a "high" in which they have incredible energy, require little sleep, and can "do anything, be anything." A more formal description follows:*

A. One or more distinct periods with a predominantly elevated expansive, or irritable mood. The elevated or irritable mood must be a prominent part of the illness and relatively persistent, although it may alternate or intermingle with depressive mood.

B. Duration of at least one week (or any duration if hospitalization is necessary), during which, for most of the time, at least three of the following symptoms have persisted (four if the mood is only irritable) and have been present to a significant degree:

   (1) increase in activity (either socially, at work, or sexually) or physical restlessness
   (2) more talkative than usual or pressure to keep talking
   (3) flight of ideas or subjective experience that thoughts are racing
   (4) inflated self-esteem (grandiosity, which may be delusional)
   (5) decreased need for sleep
   (6) distractibility, i.e., attention is too easily drawn to unimportant or irrelevant external stimuli
   (7) excessive involvement in activities that have a high potential for painful consequences which is not recognized, e.g., buying sprees, sexual indiscretions, foolish business investments, reckless driving

If these symptoms occur in the absence of schizophrenia, brain damage or drug abuse, they constitute a diagnosis of mania. Clearly, if the "high" of these patients is extreme, their behavior becomes disorganized and potentially destructive to their work as well as social and family relations.

The following case histories are presented to clarify the range of symptoms associated with mania:**

CASE I: A 24-year-old single, female copy editor was presented at a case conference two weeks after her first psychiatric hospitalization. Her admission followed an accident in which she had wrecked her car while

*Adapted from *Diagnostic and Statistical Manual of Mental Disorders,* 3rd ed. Washington, D.C.: American Psychiatric Association, 1981.

**Spitzer, R.L., Skodol, A.E., Gibbon, M., and Williams, J.B.: *DSM III Case Book.* Washington, D.C.: American Psychiatric Association, 1981.

driving at high speed late at night when she was feeling "energetic" and that "sleep was a waste of time". The episode began while she was on vacation, when she felt "high" and on the verge of a "great romance". She apparently took off all her clothes and ran naked through the woods. On the day of admission she reported hearing voices telling her that her father and the emergency room staff were emissaries of the devil, out to "get" her for no reason that she could understand.

At the case conference she was calm and cooperative and talked of the voices she had heard in the past, which she now acknowledged had not been real. She realized she had an illness, but was still somewhat irritated at being hospitalized.

CASE II: A wealthy, 72-year-old widow was referred by her children, against her will, as they thought she was becoming "senile" since the death of her husband six months previously. After the initial bereavement, which was not severe, the patient had resumed an active social life and become a volunteer at local hospitals. The family encouraged this, but over the past three months had become concerned about her going to local bars with some of the hospital staff. The referral was precipitated by her announcing her engagement to a 25-year-old male nurse, to whom she planned to turn over her house and a large amount of money. The patient's three sons, by threat and intimidation, had made her accompany them to this psychiatric evaluation. While one of her sons was talking to the psychiatrist, the patient was heard accusing the other two of trying to commit her so they could get their hands on her money.

Initially in the interview the patient was extremely angry at her sons and the psychiatrist, insisting that they couldn't understand that for the first time in her life she was doing something for herself, not for her father, her husband, or her children. She then suddenly draped herself over the couch and asked the psychiatrist if she was attractive enough to capture a 25-year-old man. She proceeded to elaborate on her fiance's physique and sexual abilities and described her life as exciting and fulfilling for the first time. She was overtalkative and repeatedly refused to allow the psychiatrist to interrupt her with questions. She said that she went out nightly with her fiance to clubs and bars and that although she did not drink, she thoroughly enjoyed the atmosphere They often went on to an after-hours place and ended up breakfasting, going to bed and making love. After only three or four hours' sleep, she would get up, feeling refreshed, and go shopping. She was spending about $700 a week on herself and giving her fiance about $500 a week, all of which she could easily afford.

The patient agreed that her behavior was unusual for someone of her age and social position, but stated she had always been conventional and now was the time to change, before it was too late. She refused to participate in formal testing, saying "I'm not going to do any stupid tests to see if I am sane". She had no obvious memory impairment and was correctly oriented in all areas. According to the family, she had no previous history of emotional disturbance.

The behaviors characteristic of mania can be controlled by lithium. There is no question that lithium is an efficacious agent and that it is effective in the vast majority of patients (Gerbino, Oleshansky, and Gershon, 1978). We have, then, a robust clinical drug response, one that we might suppose would be the object of considerable experimental interest. Oddly, this interest has been almost entirely unsystematic.

There have, of course, been a number of laboratory studies of the behavioral effects of lithium (see the review by Smith, 1977). But these have generated neither the detailed behavioral nor pharmacologic analyses needed for model development. Thus, we have a clinical phenomenon (mania) and a clinical drug response (to lithium) for which there is essentially no behavioral pharmacology. This field is an open one.

The situation is somewhat better as far as depression and its treatment are concerned because, in this case, there has been a reasonable amount of experimental study.

DEPRESSION AND THE ANTIDEPRESSANTS

The behavioral signs of depression may include psychomotor retardation or agitation, sleep disturbance, and verbal reports of a sense of worthlessness, helplessness, and hopelessness. The depressed patient may also report plans for committing suicide and, tragically, is sometimes successful in carrying them out.[1]

The following characteristics contribute to a diagnosis of depression:*

A. Dysphoric mood or loss of interest or pleasure in all or almost all usual activities and pastimes. The dysphoric mood is characterized by symptoms such as the following: depressed, sad, blue, hopeless, low, down in the dumps, or irritable. The mood disturbance must be prominent and relatively persistent but not necessarily the most dominant symptom. (For children under 6, dysphoric mood may have to be inferred from a persistently sad facial expression.)

B. At least four of the following symptoms have each been present nearly every day for a period of at least two weeks (in children under 6, at least three of the first four).

(1) poor appetite or significant weight loss (when not dieting) or in-

*Adapted from *Diagnostic and Statistical Manual of Mental Disorders,* 3rd ed. Washington, D.C.: American Psychiatric Association, 1981.

creased appetite and significant weight gain (in children under 6, failure to make expected weight gains)

(2) insomnia or hypersomnia

(3) psychomotor agitation or retardation but not merely subjective feelings of restlessness or being slowed down (in children under 6, hypoactivity)

(4) loss of interest or pleasure in usual activities, or decrease in sexual drive not limited to a period when delusional or hallucinating (in children under 6, signs of apathy)

(5) loss of energy; fatigue

(6) feelings of worthlessness, self-reproach, or excessive or inappropriate guilt (either may be delusional)

(7) complaints or evidence of diminished ability to think or concentrate, such as slowed thinking, or indecisiveness not associated with marked loosening of associations or incoherence

(8) recurrent thoughts of death or suicidal ideation, wishes to be dead, or suicide attempt

C. Neither of the following dominates the clinical picture when an affective syndrome is absent:

(1) preoccupation with a mood-incongruent delusion or hallucination

(2) bizarre behavior

D. Not superimposed on either schizophrenia, a schizophreniform disorder, or a paranoid disorder

E. Not due to an organic mental disorder or uncomplicated bereavement

The following case histories are presented to clarify the range of symptoms associated with depression:*

CASE I: The patient is a 25-year-old female graduate student in physical chemistry who was brought to the emergency room by her roommates, who found her sitting in her car with the motor running and the garage door locked. The patient had entered psychotherapy two years previously, complaining of long-standing unhappiness, feelings of inadequacy, low self-esteem, chronic tiredness, and a generally pessimistic outlook on life. While in treatment, as before, periods of well-being were limited to a few weeks at a time. During the two months before her emergency room visit

*Spitzer, R.L., Skodol, A.E., Gibbon, M. and Williams, J.B.: *DSM III Case Book*. Washington, D.C.: American Psychiatric Association, 1981.

she became increasingly depressed, developed difficulty falling asleep and trouble concentrating, and had lost ten pounds. The onset of these symptoms coincided with a rebuff she received from a chemistry laboratory instructor to whom she had become attracted.

CASE II: A 50-year-old widow was transferred to a medical center from her community mental health center, to which she had been admitted three weeks previously with severe agitation, pacing, and hand-wringing, depressed mood accompanied by severe self-reproach, insomnia, and a 6–8 kg (15 pound) weight loss. She believed that her neighbors were against her, had poisoned her coffee, and had bewitched her to punish her because of her wickedness. Seven years previously, after the death of her husband, she had required hospitalization for a similar depression, with extreme guilt, agitation, insomnia, accusatory hallucinations of voices calling her a worthless person, and preoccupation with thoughts of suicide.

THE ANTIDEPRESSANTS

There are a number of drugs that can successfully control the symptoms of depression. They fall into two major groups. The first of these are called tricyclic antidepressants, so-called because of their general chemical structure. The members of the second group are called monoamine oxidase inhibitors (MAOIs) because one of their effects is to inhibit the activity of an enzyme, monoamine oxidase (MAO). Some representatives of each of these groups is given in Table 14–1.[2]

LIMITATIONS ON THE CLINICAL DRUG RESPONSE:

The clinical phenomenon we are considering is depression, the corresponding clinical drug response is that characteristic of the antidepressants. This clinical drug response is, of course, limited by the nature of the verbal reports that define it (i.e., reports about the patients or by the patients themselves). This kind of limitation was discussed previously in the context of both the anxiolytics and the neuroleptics. We

Table 14–1

Group	Representative drugs
MAOIs	Iproniazid
	Harmaline
	Isocarboxazid
	Nialamid
Tricyclics	Imipramine
	Desipramine
	Amitriptyline
	Nortriptyline

are, again, dealing with the possible relation of one kind of behavior—verbal report—to a second kind—our laboratory model.

There are, in addition, two other kinds of limitations involved in the clinical antidepressant response: In the first place, the antidepressants in general are less consistently efficacious than lithium (in controlling mania), the neuroleptics (in controlling schizophrenia), or the anxiolytics (in controlling anxiety). Roughly 70% of patients can be expected to respond to antidepressants; the corresponding figures for lithium and the neuroleptics are about 80% and even higher for the anxiolytics. Thus, there is a less certain relationship between clinical phenomenon and drug response in the case of the antidepressants.

A second issue relates to the chronicity of treatment required for symptom control. Optimal clinical response occurs only in the course of 1 to 3 weeks of treatment with the antidepressants. This issue of chronicity will be relevant to our consideration of a laboratory model, just as it was in the case of the neuroleptics.

SECONDARY EFFECTS OF THE ANTIDEPRESSANTS

The antidepressants, like all other drugs, produce a variety of effects other than those pertinent to the clinical phenomenon for which they are prescribed. Of the many secondary effects that the antidepressants can produce, we will be concerned with two that are characteristic of the tricyclics. We will focus on these two because they are most relevant to the business of developing a model for the clinical antidepressant response.

First, the tricyclic antidepressants have sedative properties, and second, they produce anticholingergic effects. The extent to which the different tricyclics that we are considering are sedating is indicated in the second column of Table 14–2; amitriptyline is most sedating, and desipramine least, with nortriptyline and imipramine having intermediate liabilities (see Ludwig, 1980). The values in the third column indicate the relative potencies of each drug in producing anticholinergic side-effects; amitriptyline is most potent and desipramine least.

Comparison of sedative liability with anticholinergic potency reveals a general correspondence of the two effects: amitriptyline is most sedating and has the greatest anticholinergic potency; nortriptyline and imipramine are intermediate; and desipramine is least. In contrast, comparison of these effects with the approximate daily doses in the fourth column of the table shows no orderly relationship to clinical potency.

Table 14–2

Drug	Sedative liability	Anticholinergic potency*	Average daily clinical dose (potency rank)
Amitriptyline	1	1	150 (3)
Nortriptyline	2	2	75 (1)
Imipramine	2	3	150 (3)
Desipramine	3	4	100 (2)

*Adapted from Bowden, C. L., and Giffen, M. B.: *Psychopharmacology for Primary Care Physicians.* Baltimore: Williams & Wilkins, 1978.

Thus, potency in producing a clinical drug response can be dissociated from anticholinergic potency and sedative liability.

A MODEL OF THE CLINICAL ANTIDEPRESSANT RESPONSE

The antidepressants will decrease a variety of behaviors in our reference species, the laboratory rat. But this fact alone obviously does not distinguish the antidepressants from a large number of other drugs. Furthermore, the antidepressants are without selective activity in both punishment and discriminated avoidance procedures, as we have seen.[3] These facts have led to the use of a different kind of approach to developing a model. This approach involves the interaction of the antidepressants with other drugs.

The drugs chosen for this purpose are reserpine and tetrabenazine, a short-acting compound with properties equivalent to reserpine. The choice of these two is based on two facts: first, reserpine can mimic the effects of clinical depression; second, the antidepressants can antagonize this effect.

Reserpine was once widely used to control hypertension in otherwise normal patients. One of the secondary effects of reserpine used in this way is the production of frank clinical depression. In fact, before this action was fully recognized, roughly 20% of hypertensives treated with reserpine became depressed, and about 40% of these "depressed" patients were actually hospitalized for treatment (see Bunney, 1978).

This mimicry of clinical depression led to the idea that animals given reserpine (or tetrabenazine) might provide the basis for a useful laboratory model. Clearly, this idea trades on face validity. Reserpinized patients are sometimes depressed, laboratory animals given reserpine or tetrabenazine "look" depressed, and therefore it might be supposed that we have a model of depression. As we have seen, however, reliance on face validity alone can be a deceptive affair. The pertinent question is whether the antidepressants alter the effects of reserpine and tetrabenazine in ways that meet our criteria—that is, whether the antidepressants reverse the signs of laboratory "depression" (drug-induced), as they reverse the signs of clinical depression.

THE MAO INHIBITORS (MAOIs)

Early studies of the interaction of the MAOIs with reserpine indicated that these agents do reverse the depressive effects of reserpine (Squires, 1978). The many grossly observable signs of reserpine action are antagonized by pretreatment with MAOIs. This basic finding has been extended by the use of several procedures.

One such procedure, involving nondiscriminated avoidance, was described by Heise and Boff (1960). The general nature of the effects obtained with several MAOIs is shown in Figure 14–1.

The set of cumulative records in the upper portion of the Figure (A-1 and A-2) indicates that the nondiscriminated avoidance procedure maintained stable rates of responding throughout the five hours of the experimental session. (The recording pen was reset to the baseline every 15 minutes; there are 20 such periods in the record.) The effect of tetrabenazine (2.0 mg/kg) is shown in the second set of records; note that responding is eliminated about one-half hour following injection (B-1). This absence of responding is characteristic of the next 150 minutes (B-2), with some recovery occurring thereafter (B-3). (The hash marks on the record indicate the delivery of shocks.)

Pretreatment with the MAOI iproniazid reverses these effects. A dose of 40 mg/kg given 19 hours prior to the experiment resulted in an incremental, not decremental, effect of tetrabenazine (2.0 mg/kg; C-1). This increase in rate subsequently waned and was followed by a decrease (C-2) that was much shorter than that obtained with tetrabenazine alone. Recovery is shown in the bottom record (C-3).

These results were extended by McKearney (1968), who studied several schedules of positive reinforcement (FI, VI, and FR). The decremental effects of tetrabenazine on the behaviors maintained by these schedules were antagonized by MAOIs. McKearney also found that amphetamine had comparable effects. Amphetamine has not, however, been shown to be a clinically effective antidepressant. Thus, we have a hint that the procedure will generate false positives.

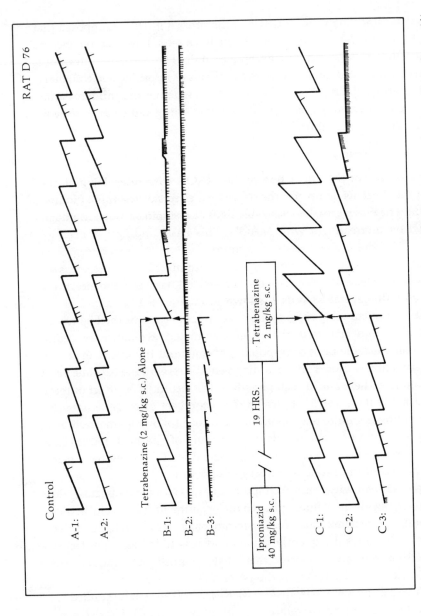

Figure 14–1. Cumulative records of responding maintained by a nondiscriminated avoidance procedure. Control rates *(A)* are decreased by tetrabenazine *(B)*; pretreatment with iproniazid *(C)* not only antagonizes this decrement but converts it to an incremental one. (Modified from Heise G.A., and Boff, E.: Behavioral determination of time and dose parameters of monoamine oxidase inhibitors. *Journal of Pharmacology and Experimental Therapeutics* 129:155–162, 1960.)

THE TRICYCLICS

We have thus far considered only antidepressants of the MAOI group. What about the tricyclics? McKearney found that at least one member of this group, imipramine, was totally lacking in antagonistic activity against tetrabenazine. It would thus seem that, in addition to false positives (amphetamine), the procedure can produce false negatives.

To make matters still more complicated, Scheckel and Boff (1964) reported data that seem to flatly contradict those reported by McKearney. In this case, several tricyclics (including imipramine) *did* antagonize the effects of tetrabenazine, whereas MAOIs did *not.* However, careful examination of these reports will show that the contradiction is more apparent than real.

As we have seen time and again, single-dose studies often mean little. But that is precisely the situation we are considering here: McKearney as well as Heise and Boff used doses of 2.0 mg/kg tetrabenazine, whereas Scheckel and Boff studied a 0.2 mg/kg dose. More to the point, Scheckel and Boff point out that the characteristic effects of the MAOIs are not obtained at doses of tetrabenazine less than 0.75 mg/kg. These relationships are summarized in Table 14–3. At first glance, these results suggest that the tricyclics are merely less potent than the MAOIs. That is, the tricyclics can antagonize the effects of low doses of tetrabenazine but lack the potency required to antagonize higher doses of tetrabenazine. But this logic does not extend to the MAOIs. If they are potent enough to antagonize *high* doses of tetrabenazine, how is it that they fail to antagonize low doses?

That question suggests that different mechanisms are involved in the antagonism of tetrabenazine by the two classes of antidepressants. Be that as it may, it is clear that tetrabenazine antagonism is a vastly complicated affair. Unfortunately, that complication is even greater than Table 14–3 implies, as we shall see as we consider the experiment by Scheckel and Boff in greater detail.

Table 14–3

Antidepressant group	Antagonism of tetrabenazine at	
	0.2mg/kg	*2.0mg/kg*
Trycyclics	Yes	No
MAOIs	No	Yes

This study involved two steps. First, the effects of a variety of drugs were each evaluated over a wide range of doses; let us call this *step 1*. Second, each of these drugs was studied in combination with tetrabenazine (0.2 mg/kg); let us call this *step 2*. The question being asked was this: Will a given drug produce an increase in responding when combined with tetrabenazine (step 2), and will it do so at a dose that is without effect when given alone (step 1)?

Scheckel and Boff found that most of the drugs that they studied failed to pass this two-step test. A partial listing is given at the left of Table 14–4. In contrast, only the tricyclic antidepressants and cocaine passed the test, as shown at the right of the table.

As already noted, the MAOIs are effective antidepressants but are ineffective with this dose of tetrabenazine. In addition, cocaine is a false positive in that clinical antidepressant activity for this drug has not been clearly demonstrated. There are even more serious complications, however. Consider the relative potencies for the tricyclics: desipramine is the most potent, nortriptyline is next, and amitriptyline and impramine follow. This ordering of potencies is very imperfectly related to the clinical values shown in Table 14–2. In particular, note that nortriptyline is clearly the most potent clinically but has an MED very nearly equal to the value for amitriptyline. All of this results in an IFE of only 25.4% ($r = 0.666$ for the MEDs in Table 16–4 and the clinical doses in Table 16–2).

Table 14–4

Negative effects	Positive effects	MED (mg/kg) For Positive Effects
Neuroleptics	Tricyclics	
Chlorpromazine	Amitriptyline	1.2
Promazine	Imipramine	1.5
	Desipramine	0.5
	Nortriptyline	1.0
Anticholinergics	Cocaine	1.7
Scopolamine		
Atropine		
Trihexyphenidyl		
Antihistamines		
Promethazine		
Phenindamine		

From Scheckel and Boff, 1964.

There is yet another complication. A patient who is clinically depressed receives medication *after* the onset of the depression; control of symptoms follows over the course of a few weeks of chronic treatment. If tetrabenazine (or reserpine) is to provide us with a model for this clinical antidepressant response, then two things should be true: first, the response to the antidepressant should occur when it is given *after* tetrabenazine; second, the antagonism of tetrabenazine should require chronic medication. The model we are considering fails on both counts: The sequence of drug administration is the wrong way around, and the effects seen are almost immediate. These facts, coupled with a low IFE, indicate that we have yet to generate an adequate model.[4]

What happens, then, when an antidepressant is given after tetrabenazine or reserpine rather than before either of them? We cannot answer this question in terms of the procedures we have been considering because the necessary data are not available. We can, however, say that the grossly observable effects of tetrabenazine or reserpine can be antagonized by subsequent injections of antidepressants. Unhappily, this fact does not help us much in developing a model: Antagonism comparable to that produced by antidepressants can also be produced by an enormous variety of other drugs, none of which have demonstrable clinical antidepressant activity. The procedure is riddled with false positives and thus fails to meet criterion A (see Hill and Tedeschi, 1971; and Squires, 1978). We thus have no model of clinical antidepressant response, at least one based on reserpine and tetrabenazine; as we shall see, however, there are other possibilities.

A SECOND MODEL OF THE CLINICAL ANTIDEPRESSANT RESPONSE

Amphetamine can increase the rate of responding maintained by nondiscriminated avoidance procedures, as we have seen. In our standard species, the rat, this effect can be dramatically augmented by pretreatment with imipramine (Carlton, 1961). Might this interaction provide us with a useful model?

The answer to that question is resoundingly negative. Augmentation can also be obtained with anticholinergics (Carlton and Didamo, 1961) as well as with a variety of other drugs in addition to the antidepressants (Scheckel and Boff, 1964). We are again confronted with an array of false positives.[5]

Although this procedure is of no use in developing a model, it is worth considering in some detail because it illustrates a vital point about studies that involve the interaction of two or more drugs.

Whenever we consider an augmentation of the effect of one drug by another, we must consider the possibility that the metabolism of the first drug, A, is inhibited by the second, B. If it is, then the combination of the two—A plus B—will produce higher levels of A, and this will amount to no more than administering higher doses of A alone. In the particular instance we are considering, the tricyclic antidepressants do inhibit the metabolism of amphetamine and thereby produce measurably higher levels of amphetamine in the brain of the rat. Thus, giving a rat an antidepressant plus amphetamine is tantamount to giving it a higher dose of amphetamine alone (Sulser, 1978).

The fact that two drugs interact in a particular way has often been used to draw inferences about the interaction of underlying physiologic mechanisms. In our example, it is known that amphetamine acts to increase the activity of certain endogenous substances in the brain; for our purposes we can call them collectively X. It is also known that the tricyclics can increase the activity of X in the brain. It thus makes perfect sense to suppose that the tricyclics augment the behavioral effects of amphetamine because of a common action on X. But this conclusion is obviously unwarranted if the tricyclics retard the metabolism of amphetamine to produce functionally higher levels of amphetamine. In fact, in those species in which the tricyclics do not retard amphetamine metabolism, the augmentation of behavioral effect is not obtained.

Although the interaction of amphetamine with the tricyclics thus fails to provide us with a model, it does provide us with an important rule: In any study of the interactions of different drugs, the prospect of altered metabolism must be examined. If it is not, totally inaccurate interpretations of the augmentation may result.[6]

A THIRD MODEL OF THE CLINICAL ANTIDEPRESSANT RESPONSE

We have thus far failed to develop a satisfactory model of the clinical antidepressant response. There is, however, another way of approaching the issue, one involving a phenomenon called **helplessness.**

As described by Seligman (1975), the basic procedure for the induction of helplessness involves two stages. In the first of these (I), animals are exposed to a situation in which responding is irrelevant to outcome, in which responding is not linked to reinforcement. In the second (II), the performance of the animals is evaluated in a situation in which responding *is* relevant to outcome, in which reinforcement is contingent on responding. Thus, for example, animals that first receive inescapable electric shock (I) are then tested for their ability to learn to avoid electric shock (II). The performance of these experimental animals in stage II is compared to the performance of controls that have not undergone stage I. The result of this comparison is that the performance of the experimental animals is vastly inferior to that of the controls.

Seligman has also indicated that this effect is not restricted to stimuli such as electric shock. That is, animals that are given positive reinforcement (e.g., food pellets) in a situation in which these reinforcements are independent of responding (stage I) also become "helpless" in that they show deficits in learning to respond for reinforcement in a subsequent test (stage II).

Seligman has suggested that the experimental animals learn that responding is "futile" in stage I, and that they are therefore helpless in stage II. It is this helplessness that may provide a model of depression. Seligman has described the relationship in this way:

Learned helplessness is caused by learning that responding is independent of reinforcement; so the model suggests that the cause of depression is the belief that action is futile.

Seligman has bolstered the presumed relation of helplessness to depression by enumerating a number of functional parallels in which the phenomena seen experimentally do seem to correspond to those seen clinically (see also Huesmann, 1978). Furthermore, the phenomenon can be obtained in a variety of species, including humans. It may therefore be that helplessness can provide us with a model of clinical antidepressant response. That is, antidepressants might be expected to antagonize helplessness and therefore to reduce the performance deficits seen in stage II.

An experiment by Leshner, Remler, Biegon, and Samuel (1979) addressed this issue. In this study, laboratory rats were given a series of inescapable electric shocks (stage I) and were then given a series of injections prior to a test in which they could escape shock (stage II). Other animals received injections prior to stage II but had not undergone stage I.

The injections were either saline or desipramine at one of two dose levels. These injections were given immediately after stage I and once a day for a week thereafter. The procedure was thus unlike those we have been considering in that the effects of chronic, not acute, medication were evaluated.

Animals that had not been shocked in stage I and had been given saline required about 15 seconds to escape in stage II. Furthermore, other unshocked animals that were given either 10.0 or 20.0 mg/kg of desipramine required about the same amount of time to escape shock in this stage. There was, then, no effect of drug in the absence of shock in stage I. In contrast, the animals that were given shock in stage I but no drug required more time in stage II (26.3 seconds), presumably because they were helpless. If helplessness amounts to depression, then desipramine should antagonize this effect. That it did so is shown by the data in Table 14–5. The animals given shock in stage I but no drug treatment took, relative to controls, about 11 additional seconds to escape (the third column in Table 14–5). Desipramine reduced this effect in a dose-dependent manner. There is thus an indication that an antidepressant can antagonize a presumptive analog of clinical depression.

But is this result any more than suggestive? Unfortunately, it is not; the study by Leshner and his coworkers is important but certainly not definitive, for several reasons. In the first place, we do not know what the effects of a single administration of desipramine might be because only chronic treatments were studied. If single injections were effective, the relevance to clinical drug response would be reduced, as we have already noted. Furthermore, we do not know whether desipramine might alter the sensitivity to electric shock.[7]

More important than these considerations, however, is the fact that the procedure studied only one drug at only two dose levels. This means that the phenomena at hand cannot be evaluated with regard to criterion B, and at a more elementary level, there is no way of knowing whether the procedure is a discriminating one—whether it satisfies cri-

Table 14–5

Dose (mg/kg)*	Time to escape in stage II	Difference from control (= 15.0)
0	26.3	11.3
10	19.6	4.6
20	16.6	1.6

*Given daily for 8 days; animals were given shock in stage I.
Adapted from Leshner, Remler, Biegon, and Samuel, 1979.

terion A. Furthermore, in relation to the issue of criterion A, the possible effects of the anticholinergics are important. Our concern here, after all, is a suppression of behavior in stage II—and we know that the anticholinergics can antagonize suppression in many, although not all, experimental situations (see Anisman, 1978; and Anisman, Remington, and Sklar, 1979). We have already seen (see Note 5) that the antidepressants do have substantial anticholinergic activity but that the anticholinergics lack clinical antidepressant activity.[8]

As far as these data are concerned, then, there is no way of evaluating the possibility that the phenomenon could form the basis of a model for the clinical antidepressant response. We can, nonetheless, look at the idea of helplessness in other ways. These approaches do not involve the stage I–stage II procedure just discussed, but they do have a general correspondence to the basic idea. Might they therefore help us to generate a model?

A VARIANT ON HELPLESSNESS

Let us now consider a variation on the procedure used by Leshner and his coworkers. Recall that their technique involved (1) stage I (to induce helplessness, a presumptive analog of depression), (2) drug treatment (analogous to clinical intervention), and (3) stage II (a test for drug effect). In the variant examined here, Sherman, Ahlers, Petty, and Henn (1979) gave drug treatments *before* stage I, not after it.

Sherman and his coworkers found that chronic, but not acute, pretreatment with one antidepressant, imipramine, produced a dose-dependent antagonism of stage II deficits in escape responding. There is thus a parallel to the effects reported by Leshner and colleagues in that chronic antidepressant treatment antagonized response deficits (see Table 14–5). In addition, the finding that acute treatment was without effect points to an important correspondence with clinical findings (criterion C).

This study also involved an examination of an anxiolytic, lorazepam. This drug antagonized stage II deficits following acute treatment but not following chronic treatment. (The findings with lorazepam were thus complementary to those with imipramine.) In addition, the neuroleptic chlorpromazine was found to be without effect following either an acute or a chronic dose regimen.

There is again a suggestion that differentiation among drug classes is possible. Unfortunately, however, the essential dose–response information on lorazepam and chlorpromazine is not available, nor are there

data on a broad range of other drugs including the MAOIs and anticholinergics. Furthermore, these studies have failed to incorporate an examination of the possible role of analgesia (see Note 7).

Another feature of these data is also troubling. Recall that all drug
treatments were given before the stage I–stage II sequence. If the effects
of stage I are to be taken as an analog of clinical depression, then the
data at hand indicate that imipramine would be useful in *preventing* depression.

The available clinical information does, in fact, indicate that the antidepressants do have at least some prophylactic effects (Kessler, 1978).
But this fact does not help us with our main problem of developing a
model for the reversal of already developed depression by the antidepressants. That is, the important findings of Sherman and his coworkers
are based on a paradigm that involves drug–stage I–stage II. We need
data based on a paradigm that involves stage I–drug–stage II if our
model of clinical drug response is to be pertinent to the major way in
which antidepressants are used in clinical practice.

A SECOND VARIANT ON HELPLESSNESS

The essence of helplessness lies in the fact that responding has no relationship to the occurrence of stimuli, whether these be electric shocks
or positive reinforcements like food. We will consider two other procedures that involve such response-independent stimuli. One of these is
the now-familiar CER procedure; the other is a response-independent
reinforcement procedure developed by Miczek (1973a). (Miczek's experiment will be discussed in greater detail in Chapter 15.)

The procedure studied by Miczek involved presenting a stimulus, the
termination of which was coincident with the delivery of a food pellet
regardless of whether the animal had responded. Thus, the technique
is analogous to the CER in that events coincident with stimulus termination are response-independent; shock delivery coincides with stimulus termination in the case of the CER, whereas a "free" reinforcement
coincides with termination in the Miczek procedure.*

Reinforcements (food or shock) are independent of responding in
both of these procedures, and animals fail to respond during the stimuli
that precede reinforcement in both. There are, therefore, behavioral deficits analogous to those seen in stage II of the usual helplessness procedure. These instances of a failure to respond might, on the face of it,

*The Miczek technique is similar to one of those used to develop helplessness; see Selig-
man (1975), p. 34.

be supposed to correspond to the absence of behavior characteristic of clinical depression. That is, in both instances, the animals seem to "give up" in the face of response-independent stimuli.

Unfortunately, there is no evidence indicating that the antidepressants antagonize these behavioral deficits. We do know, however, that Miczek found that chlordiazepoxide (but not amphetamine) antagonized the behavioral suppression seen in the CER procedure, whereas amphetamine (but not chlordiazepoxide) antagonized the suppression engendered by response-independent food reinforcement. There is, therefore, a pharmacologic differentiation of the behaviors that does not correspond to the idea that they represent the effects of a common process that controls helplessness. Furthermore, even if we were to regard either of these two phenomena as instances of helplessness, we would immediately be confronted by two clear false positives: Neither chlordiazepoxide nor amphetamine has clinical antidepressant activity.[9]

A THIRD VARIANT ON HELPLESSNESS

Another procedure that has been extensively used for the study of a broad range of drugs is one that engenders a phenomenon called **behavioral despair.**

In experiments using this procedure (Porsolt, Bertin, and Jalfre, 1977; Porsolt, Anton, Blavet, and Jalfre, 1978), rats or mice are placed in a container filled with water. They at first swim vigorously and, then, after about two minutes, their swimming subsides to be replaced by periods of immobility of increasing duration. During these periods, the animals float passively with their heads just above water level. After about four minutes of immersion, swimming is almost completely absent and the animals are immobile about 85% of the time. Apparently the animals, literally plunged into an inescapable situation, simply "give up"—hence, the term *despair.* Furthermore, the idea of despair has an obvious conceptual linkage to ideas of futility and helplessness. Seligman has, in fact, implied a continuity of despair and helplessness in his discussion of early experiments by Richter.* But do these suggestions about the relation of despair and helplessness to depression provide a model of clinical antidepressant response?

We can begin to get at this question by determining whether the antidepressants antagonize immobility, the presumed indicant of depression. Porsolt and his coworkers have shown that a broad range of an-

*See Seligman (1975), pp. 169ff.

tidepressants do, in fact, reduce immobility. So far, unlike the experimental animals, we are on solid ground.

But what about the effects of other drugs that are not antidepressants? Does the procedure meet criterion A? It does not. Amphetamine, caffeine, pentobarbital, several antihistamines, and several anticholinergics have all been found to reduce immobility (Browne, 1979; Schecter and Chance, 1979; Wallach and Hedley, 1979). We are again confronted with an impressive array of false positives. We must once more conclude that we do not have a satisfactory model of clinical antidepressant response.

FACE VALIDITY AND EMPIRICAL VALIDATION

All of the procedures that we have considered involve an admittedly persuasive kind of face validity. It is true that reserpine and tetrabenazine seem to mimic the signs of clinical depression; it is true that the phenomenon of helplessness and its variants have an appealing parallel to depression. Intuition alone would suggest that, on the face of it, these procedures should have provided satisfactory models—yet they have not done so. Thus, if we had been content to rely on face validity alone, we could have been seriously misled, as our examination of the criteria for empirical validation has made clear. This is the important lesson to be learned here.

This is not to say that these procedures will never lead us to a useful model.[10] Rather, it is to say that, appearances notwithstanding, they have not yet done so. Thus, because we do not have a satisfactory model, the elucidation of the mechanisms that may control the clinical antidepressant response is necessarily at a standstill.[11]

NOTES

1. Many depressed patients have a history of manic or near-manic (hypomania) episodes; they are referred to as *bipolar depressives. Unipolar depressives,* on the other hand, are characterized by episodes of depression without precedent periods of mania or hypomania. It appears that, if lithium is given to bipolar patients during their manic episodes and if this medication is maintained into the subsequent period of normality, the recurrent episodes of depression can be eliminated, at least in some patients. In this sense, lithium can be viewed as an antidepressant.

2. A large number of antidepressants is currently available. Unfortunately, systematic data of the kind we need are not also available. We will, therefore, be forced to restrict our consideration to a relatively few drugs. This restricted range is nonetheless sufficient to highlight the deficiencies of the various candidates for laboratory models that will be discussed.

3. In contrast to the effects seen in the laboratory rat, tricyclic antidepressants can produce marked increases in the responding of pigeons. Increases in responding by pigeons have also been found with chlorpromazine, a finding that may be due to the similarity in the chemical structures of chlorpromazine and the tricyclic antidepressants.

4. It could be assumed, of course, that whatever changes are required for an antidepressant effect in humans are somehow not required in rats. Thus, the effects of antidepressants might be expected to be delayed in the former and immediate in the latter. This assumption would require, however, an explicit demonstration of such differential effects in the two species if it is to amount to more than merely begging the question.

5. There have been occasional claims for antidepressant activity due to the anticholinergics; none of these has been adequately documented. On the other hand, the tricyclics do have substantial anticholinergic activity. Thus, it is important to examine explicitly the effects of the anticholinergics in any proposed model.

6. Suppose that a drug procedures a decremental effect when given alone but produces an incremental effect when given with another. Neither an increase nor a decrease in rate of metabolism can directly account for this result. That is, increased metabolism would result in functionally less drug availability and a reduced decremental effect but not an incremental one; decreased metabolism would result in functionally greater drug availability and a greater decremental effect. Effects like those shown in Figure 14–1 cannot, therefore, be attributed to an altered metabolism of the kind considered here.

7. It has been reported that prior electric shock in stage I can produce analgesia during the period when stage II would take place (Maier and Coon, 1979). Analgesia during stage II testing could, of course, reduce the tendency to respond and thereby produce a response decrement independently of the role of a presumed process of helplessness. Furthermore, if drugs attenuated the analgesic process, they would appear to attenuate helplessness. Thus, an explicit ex-

amination of the possible role of analgesia is crucial to the development of a model. Unfortunately, such a role has not been consistently evaluated in the experiments discussed here.

8. Aramine is a drug that has been reported to disrupt helplessness (Harrell, Haynes, Lambert, and Sininger, 1978). Aramine presumably does not enter the brain and, in any case, has not been shown to have clinical antidepressant activity.

9. These data do not, of course, preclude the possibility that chronically administered antidepressants may antagonize the suppression engendered by either or both of the procedures.

10. In fact, it seems likely that useful models will evolve from the procedures studied by Leshner and his coworkers and by Sherman and colleagues. Other promising approaches to the problem have been discussed by Cairncross, Cos, Forster, and Wren (1978) and by Katz (1981).

11. There have been indications (McGuire and Seiden, 1980) that tricyclic antidepressants uniquely lengthen the interresponse times characteristic of DRL schedules at doses that do not also produce an overall decrement in responding. This effect is totally devoid of face validity yet could meet all of our criteria. Future research will tell the tale.

Section 6
The Analysis of Models

IN SECTION IV, we were confronted with the problem of diversity, a problem that led us directly to a consideration of classification as a means of ordering information. The system of classification that we chose to use led, in turn, to the business of developing models of clinical drug response. As we have now seen, we have had only limited success in that undertaking; however, we have made other gains along the way.

First, we certainly have a clearer understanding of how models can be evolved. Second, we have seen how the process of model development can be used to organize a large body of data irrespective of their success in providing us with a model. In the case of the antidepressants, for example, we have been able to systematize a wide range of drug effects even though we have only suggestions for future model development that are, at best, provocative. Third, we are now in a position to take the next step—to analyze those models that have proven to be reasonably satisfactory. Thus, we will focus on the anxiolytics and neuroleptics; we will, perforce, leave the antidepressants and lithium behind.

Our analysis of these models will take place on two levels. At the first level, we will address the question of why it is that the models work as well as they do. As we shall see, our analysis of the anxiolytic response (Chapter 15) will lead us to an interpretation of the clinical phenomenon upon which it is based. That is, we will be able to place what we have learned in the laboratory into a clinical context. On the other hand, a parallel analysis of the neuroleptic response (Chapter 16) will make it clear that our model is even less satisfactory than it now appears to be.

The second level of analysis will bring us back to the issue with which we began our consideration of models of clinical drug response. The ultimate but not exclusive use of a model is to elucidate the physiologic mechanisms that underlie the fact of classification. Just as the grouping of elements partly rests on an underlying communality in atomic structure, so too must a grouping of drugs at least partly rest on an underlying communality in physiologic process. Chapter 17 will be devoted to a discussion of how models can be used to elucidate what those processes may be. In Chapter 18, we will conclude with an overview of this second kind of analysis.

Chapter 15

The Anxiolytic Response

OUR MODEL OF the clinical anxiolytic response is a reasonably satisfactory one. Why should the model meet the four criteria as well as it actually does? That is, what variables underlie the fact that our model can be reasonably well validated?

PROCEDURAL SPECIFICITY

Our model of clinical response for the anxiolytics is based on the low rates of responding induced by electric shock.[1] Might *any* procedure involving electric shock also provide useful models of the clinical anxiolytic activity? Furthermore, are the low rates that are sensitive to anxiolytics dependent on shock, or might any low-rate behavior also generate a useful model? Let us first consider each of three procedures involving shock—discriminated avoidance, nondiscriminated avoidance, and the CER—in terms of their usefulness in evaluating the clinical anxiolytic response.

Discriminated Avoidance Anxiolytics do decrease discriminated avoidance behavior, but as we saw in Chapter 13, they do not do so in a specific way. That is, doses of anxiolytics that decrease avoidance responding also produce deficits in escape behavior. But such nonspecificity is characteristic of an enormous range of drugs, none of which is clinically anxiolytic. Thus, discriminated avoidance procedures fail to meet criterion A.

Nondiscriminated Avoidance   Similar problems with specificity pertain to nondiscriminated avoidance but in a more refined way. Anxiolytics have been reported to disrupt nondiscriminated avoidance responding in complex ways (see Heise and Boff, 1962; and Zbinden and Randall, 1967). It turns out that, within a broad spectrum of drugs, it is not possible to distinguish anxiolytics from neuroleptics. We will have more to say about these data in the next chapter; as we will see, the procedure also generates unequivocal false negatives.[2] Nondiscriminated avoidance, like discriminated avoidance, therefore fails to meet criterion A.

CER   Recall that the CER is a technique that, like punishment, involves low rates of responding due to electric shock. The fundamental difference in procedures is that punishment involves response-contingent shock whereas the CER involves shock delivered independently of the animal's behavior.

The low rates obtained in the CER paradigm can be increased by the anxiolytic drugs, but these effects are not consistent (see Millenson and Leslie, 1974; Bignami, 1978). Furthermore, conclusions about the CER must be limited by the fact that it has not been systematically evaluated as a model of clinical anxiolytic response. The data pertinent to criterion B are not available because a single procedure has not been used to evaluate an array of drugs over a range of doses. We are therefore forced to put the CER aside because of a lack of relevant information.[3]

LOW RESPONSE RATES

The data we have thus far considered indicate that shock-dependent behaviors are not uniquely sensitive to the anxiolytics. That brings us to the question of whether low rates induced by means other than shock might be selectively sensitive to the anxiolytics. We can begin to consider this issue by examining an experiment by Miczek (1973a).

This experiment involved a novel technique for engendering low rates. Animals were trained to respond on a VI schedule into which a signal was inserted. Coincident with the termination of this signal the animals received a single reinforcement that was delivered *independently* of responding. Thus, these "free" reinforcements were not contingent on responding; as a result, response rates were very low during the signals. (See the discussion of helplessness in Chapter 14.)

Miczek found that chlordiazepoxide was almost entirely devoid of a rate-increasing effect in this situation. These low rates were not, however, totally insensitive to drug action; amphetamine produced a profound, dose-dependent increase.

This generalization was extended to yet another study by Miczek (1973b). In this case, responding was maintained by a multiple schedule involving three components: the first, a VI schedule; the second, a punishment schedule; and the third, a period in which no responses were reinforced. The experimental arrangement thus allowed for a direct comparison of two means of producing low response rates—punishment and nonreinforcement. The results of comparisons involving amphetamine and chlordiazepoxide are shown in Figure 15–1.

As the panel at the top of Figure 15–1 makes clear, amphetamine increases the low rates controlled by nonreinforcement, whereas it has little effect on the low rates controlled by punishment (see Table 12–3). In contrast, chlordiazepoxide (in the bottom panel) has a complementary effect: low rates due to punishment are increased (see Table 12–2), whereas there is only a minor effect on responding in the absence of reinforcement.

These and a variety of other data indicate that procedures that involve shock (but not low rates due to punishment) are not selectively sensitive to the anxiolytics. Similarly, procedures that involve low rates (but not punishment) are not selectively sensitive to the anxiolytics. The key to selectivity thus lies in procedures that involve punishment; this, of course, is precisely what our model does involve.

SECONDARY CLINICAL EFFECTS

The anxiolytics are sedative, as we have seen. This property is, in fact, their only secondary effect of behavioral consequence.

It has been argued that the action of these drugs inheres in their sedative effects rather than in any specific anxiety reduction they produce. If that were true, however, any drug with sedative properties would also be anxiolytic. At a clinical level we know that antihistamines as well as a number of neuroleptics and antidepressants are sedative; yet they have not been shown to be specifically anxiolytic. Furthermore, these same drugs are ineffective in our model.

It is true that anxiolytics can be sedating, but it is not true that all sedatives are anxiolytics. Thus, the reports of anxiety reduction that characterize the anxiolytics cannot be referred to their sedative properties alone.[4]

We also know that the anxiolytics are muscle relaxants (i.e., they pro-

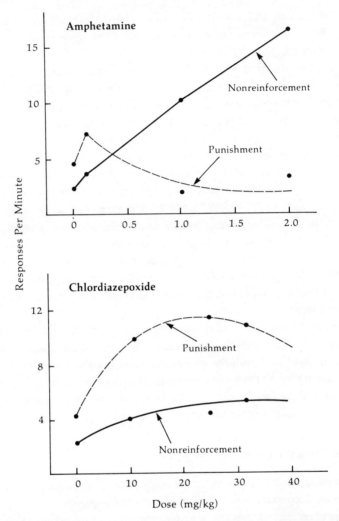

Figure 15–1. Dose–response functions describing the effects of amphetamine (top) and chlordiazepoxide (bottom) on the low rates maintained by punishment or nonreinforcement procedures. (Values estimated from published figures in Miczek, K. A.: Effects of scopolamine, amphetamine and chlordiazepoxide on punishment. *Psychopharmacologia (Berlin)* 28:373–389, 1973.)

duce a reduction in the tension that can be directly recorded from muscles.) It might, therefore, be supposed that it is this property that underlies anxiety reduction.

If that were true, all muscle relaxants would be anxiolytic but they are not. Drugs such as mephenesin, carisoprodol, chlorzoxazone, and metaxalone all have muscle relaxant properties (and are sedating), but their clinical anxiolytic activity has not been clearly established. Furthermore, they do not increase punished responding (see Lippa, Nash, and Greenblatt, 1979).

These conclusions do not mean, however, that sedation and muscle relaxation are totally irrelevant to the clinical anxiolytic response. It is reasonable to suppose that these activities do supplement the more fundamental anxiety reduction that is characteristic of the anxiolytics. That is, sedation and muscle relaxation may interact with anxiolysis to produce the clinical response, but these two alone are not sufficient.[5]

SECONDARY LABORATORY EFFECTS

When we consider our model in detail, it becomes obvious that the effects we have been considering could occur if the anxiolytics either (1) increased motivation for food reinforcement or (2) decreased the efficacy of electric shock. That is, if the anxiolytics mimicked the effects of food deprivation, the resultant increase in motivation might be expected to increase responding. Alternatively, if the anxiolytics produced analgesia, an increase in responding might also be expected.

INCREASED MOTIVATION

There is no doubt that the anxiolytics can mimic a variety of the effects of food deprivation, as described by Wise and Dawson (1974). These agents therefore produce increased food intake in laboratory animals and humans. It is not true, however, that increased food deprivation, even to extreme levels, can mimic the effects of the anxiolytics in punishment situations. Furthermore, as Wise and Dawson point out, the anxiolytics do not mimic the effects of water deprivation. It is therefore significant that water reinforcement, rather than food, can be used without any fundamental alteration in the effects of the anxiolytics on punished behavior (see Sepinwall and Cook, 1978). The plausible idea about a role of increased motivation is not, therefore, supported by the available data.

ANALGESIA

Induction of analgesia might be expected to increase punished responding. If this were the case, however, morphine should certainly increase responding; but it does not consistently do so, as we have already seen. Furthermore, anxiolytics do not have analgesic activity in tests where drugs such as morphine unquestionably do. Finally, consider the effects of discontinuing shock entirely. Such a condition is tantamount to perfect analgesia—"no shock, no pain." But when shock is discontinued, animals do not immediately begin responding; rather, low rates are maintained for protracted periods even in the absence of shock. Thus, we can comfortably reject the idea that analgesia is a critical factor in producing the effects of the anxiolytics in our model (again, see Sepinwall and Cook, 1978).

OTHER LABORATORY EFFECTS

The prospect that increased motivation or analgesia could account for increased rates is certainly a plausible idea, albeit an inadequate one. Equally plausible is the idea that the effects of the anxiolytics can be attributed to rate-dependency or stimulus change.

RATE-DEPENDENCY

It is certainly reasonable to suppose that, in keeping with the low rates due to punishment, the effects of the anxiolytics could be an instance of rate-dependency. If this were the case, however, we would expect that our criteria for the anxiolytic response would be met in a wide range of situations. But as we have seen, there is a procedural specificity in the effects of the anxiolytics. In addition, the anxiolytics can antagonize punishment-induced suppression independently of rate-dependency (see Figure 4–6, A).

Furthermore, one drug that unequivocally demonstrates rate-dependency is amphetamine. But amphetamine is uniformly ineffective in increasing responding suppressed by punishment, as noted in Table 10–3. It does, however, increase the low rates seen with other procedures.

This is not to say, however, that the effects of the anxiolytics are immune to rate-dependency. The anxiolytics can, in fact, produce rate-dependent effects in a variety of situations. But as far as our model is concerned, the characteristic sign of anxiolytic activity cannot be accounted for in this way (see Sanger and Blackman, 1976; 1981).

STIMULUS CHANGE

In our model, animals are trained in the absence of drug and then tested with drug. Because drugs can act as stimuli, it might be supposed that the change in stimulus conditions (no drug–drug) produces a disruption so that low rates are increased (see Chapter 7).

However, attributing this loss of suppression to stimulus change would not explain why there is both a procedural and a pharmacologic specificity in the effects of the anxiolytics. That is, there is no reason to suppose that stimulus change would be uniquely relevant to certain drugs (the anxiolytics) only when they are evaluated with certain procedures (punishment). Thus, stimulus change certainly may be involved in mediating some of the effects of the anxiolytics, but it just as certainly cannot explain all of their effects in punishment procedures. At a more general level, stimulus change—and the rate-dependency it may produce (see Figure 7–2)—are nonspecific effects. They cannot, therefore, fully account for the pharmacologic and behavioral specificity characteristic of punishment procedures.

INTERPRETING THE MODEL

If none of the factors just considered—stimulus change, rate-dependency, analgesia, increased motivation, or sedation—can account for the specificity in our model, what can?

The fact that our model does meet the various criteria we have considered cannot be due solely to the fact that it induces low response rates, nor can it be due solely to the fact that it involves shock. Rather, the response contingency must embody two consequences: (1) responding is reinforced, but (2) it is also punished. There is a kind of duality in that a single response may have a positive or a negative outcome, or both.

This arrangement can be described as a *conflict* situation. The usage does not, however, mean that the animal is in a *state* of conflict (see Chapter 12, Note 3). As we have seen, we can never be certain about such states even though they may actually occur in laboratory animals and in humans. The idea of conflict does, nonetheless, lead us to a specification of an environmental contingency for the anxiolytic response: Contingencies in which responding can have both a reinforcing and an aversive outcome set the occasion for the anxiolytic response.[6]

THE CLINICAL PHENOMENON AND THE MODEL

The formulation we are considering brings us to a consideration of the relationship of the clinical *phenomenon* of anxiety to our model. Table 15–1 clarifies this relationship. The clinical phenomenon (entry I) with which we have been concerned is surely due to a multiplicity of factors. These are denoted as A, B, C, and so forth. We know that the anxiolytics must antagonize at least one of these factors. This antagonism is sym-

Table 15–1

I. Clinical phenomenon	II. Clinical drug response
Verbal reports of anxiety (A, B, C . . .)	Verbal reports of reduced anxiety (A', D, E . . .)
III. Laboratory phenomenon	IV. Laboratory drug response
Suppression and reinforcement loss (A, H, I . . .)	Reduced suppression and reinforcement gain (A', F, G . . .)

bolized as A' in entry II. (Note that the clinical drug response is also controlled by other factors that may be independent of those controlling the clinical phenomenon.)

We also know that some element in the clinical drug response must be involved in the laboratory drug response (entry IV). If this were not the case, our model could not satisfy the various criteria we have used in evaluating it. Thus, A' appears in both entries II and IV.

Because A' is a factor in the laboratory drug response, its complement, A, must be a factor in the laboratory phenomenon (entry III). (Again, factors other than A and A' are involved in III and IV).

When we take a clockwise tour around Table 15–2, we move from I to II, from II to IV, from IV to III and, necessarily, back to I again. In other words, the environmental contingency just described must be a determining factor not only of the laboratory phenomenon but of the clinical phenomenon as well.

The idea that this tour generates cannot, however, be regarded as a blinding new clinical insight. Indeed, the idea that such a contingency is a factor in producing reports of anxiety is an old one. What is new is the following. Our analysis focuses not on a state of the organism but on an environmental contingency that, first, defines a factor in clinical anxiety that, second, is modified by the anxiolytics. The following three ordinary examples illustrate the point.

Consider the prospect of taking an examination of some sort. This prospect is certainly one of the most common sources of reported anxiety, and it is one that embodies the contingency just discussed. Taking the test involves the opportunity to pass (be reinforced) or to fail (be punished). The contingency can, of course, be avoided entirely. Not taking the exam at all, however, means certain failure. Thus, most people do take examinations but report being anxious about them.

Consider gambling. The decision to gamble may be followed by loss (punishment), but *not* gambling prevents the opportunity of winning (reinforcement). In fact, many people report that they enjoy the "tension" of gambling, whereas others report that they rarely gamble because the activity is too anxiety-provoking. It is probably not coincidental, therefore, that the gambling experiments discussed in Chapter 12 engender behavior that is sensitive to the anxiolytics.

Finally, consider the common fear of flying. Not taking the plane will result in a loss of those reinforcements that initiated the motivation to travel in the first place. But flight may be severely punished, because accidents do occur.

It is, of course, absurd to suppose that the environment contingency involved in these and other instances of reported anxiety can account for all the complex phenomena seen clinically. We do not know, for example, why some people report that certain contingencies are anxiety-provoking and others are not. And we certainly do not know why a few people find so many situations anxiety-provoking and why they are unable to cope with them realistically. (It is the lack of realistic coping, in fact, that defines "neurotic anxiety.")

But this is not the main point. The point is, rather, that our model dictates an environment contingency, and that this contingency makes sense in light of what is known about clinical anxiety and the anxiolytics. The model has, then, a kind of face validity. Its plausibility does not, however, depend in any way upon such validity. The face validity that the model does have is a bonus, but the validation itself is entirely empirical.[7]

NOTES

1. File and Hyde (1979) have reported on an interesting and potentially useful approach to developing a different kind of model of the anxiolytic response. Whether it will ultimately meet our criteria remains to be seen; also see the article by Iversen (1980).

2. It is important to bear in mind that, although our model does generate a few equivocal false positives, it does not generate false negatives.

3. Rawlins, Feldon, Salmon, Gray, and Garrud (1980) have reported experiments indicating that the CER is not as insensitive to anxiolytic activity as it is generally thought to be. If, however, the CER is to be given serious consideration as a model, the bases of various inconsistencies, false positives, and false negatives will have to be clarified (see Bignami, 1978).

4. Sedation does appear to be an important adjunctive effect in some patients. That is, some but certainly not all patients are more likely to report on a reduction in anxiety if they also report that the drug produces sedation (see Rickels, Downing, and Winokur, 1978).

5. Anxiolytics are, as we have noted, also anticonvulsants. As a consequence, they can antagonize convulsions induced by other drugs. In fact, the potencies of different anxiolytics in antagonizing convulsions induced by one drug, pentylenetatrazol, correlates well with the median clinical potencies of these same anxiolytics. (Lippa and coworkers (1979) reported an r of 0.793 for nine anxiolytics; IFE = 39.1%, a value substantially lower than that obtained with our model.) However, other anticonvulsants, the hydantoins, have not been shown to be anxiolytic. Thus, anticonvulsant activity per se is not linked to anxiolytic activity.

6. One of the important relationships in Table 10–3 is the parallelism in the effects of the three different drugs on FR and punished behavior. There is a suggestion, therefore, that FR responding could provide a useful laboratory model of the clinical aniolytic response.

Of particular interest is the general finding that the post-reinforcement pauses in FR are shortened by one anxiolytic, pentobarbital; this attenuation is the major reason why there are overall increases in response rates, as indicated by the (+) entries at 2 in Table 10–3. Also note that FR, like punished responding, is insensitive to the rate-increasing effects of amphetamine and shows only decremental effects following chlorpromazine. These parallels suggest that the low rates controlled by reinforcement in FR share functional properties with those low rates induced by punishment based on electric shock. At the very least, they illustrate the potential value of a classificatory system in that, with such a system, parallels amenable to further investigation emerge.

7. It should be possible to identify specific reinforcement–punishment contingencies relevant to different patients and then to determine the extent to which their reported anxiety is reduced by the anxiolytics in the face of these contingencies.

Chapter 16
The Neuroleptic Response

OUR MODEL OF the clinical neuroleptic response is less satisfactory than the one we have developed for the anxiolytics. We should, nonetheless, consider its properties because, in doing so, we can highlight some of the general problems intrinsic to the use of models.

We can approach these problems in the same way that we analyzed the anxiolytic response in the previous chapter. Thus, we begin by addressing the question of procedural specificity.

PROCEDURAL SPECIFICITY

The fact that discriminated avoidance is selectively sensitive to the neuroleptics cannot inhere solely in the fact that it involves shock. If this were true, then all other procedures involving shock would be selective as well—but, as we have seen, they surely are not.

The selectivity also does not inhere in an avoidance contingency per se. If this were true, then *non*discriminated avoidance would be selectively sensitive to the neuroleptics. It is true that the neuroleptics can decrease nondiscriminated avoidance responding, but this effect does not differentiate them from other drugs, as shown in Table 16–1.

NONDISCRIMINATED AVOIDANCE

Heise and Boff (1962) reported that all of the drugs they studied decreased rates of nondiscriminated avoidance responding. As a consequence, all necessarily increased the numbers of shocks received; the MEDs at which these increases occurred are given in the middle column of Table 16–1.

Heise and Boff also reported "escape failure/shock" ratios (given in the right-hand column). These ratios were obtained by comparing two values: the MED at which escape *failure* occurred and the MED at which shocks were increased. Thus, a drug could produce a shock increase at some MED but produce an escape failure only at a higher MED. Such drugs would, therefore, produce ratios greater than 1.0. On the other hand, if a drug produced a shock increase at some MED, and if the animals also failed to escape at this dose, then this nonspecific effect would produce a ratio of about 1.0.

The neuroleptics do produce high ratios, just as they do in discriminated avoidance—but so do most anxiolytics. The range of ratios for the anxiolytics is 1.0–5.5; this range overlaps that for the neuroleptics. Equally striking are findings that the ratios for chlorpromazine and chlordiazepoxide are almost identical and that diazepam is less potent (MED = 10.0) than chlordiazepoxide (MED = 4.2) in increasing shocks. (Note, however, that morphine has a ratio comparable to the neuroleptics, just as it does in discriminated avoidance.)

These and similar data make it clear that the selective sensitivity obtained with discriminated avoidance is not contingent on the use of shock avoidance per se. It thus appears that differential sensitivity to

Table 16–1*

	MED** shock increase	MED escape failure/ MED shock increase
Neuroleptics		
Chlorpromazine	0.21	3.4
Trifluoperazine	0.03	1.9
Chlorprothixene	0.18	1.7
Anxiolytics		
Diazepam	10.00	5.5
Chlordiazepoxide	4.20	3.8
Phenobarbital	30.00	2.1
Meprobamate	103.00	1.0
Analgesics		
Morphine	0.75	2.7

*Data from Heise, G. A., and Boff, E.: Continuous avoidance as a base-line for measuring behavioral effects of drugs. *Psychopharmacologia (Berlin)* 3: 264–282, 1962.
**MEDs are in mg/kg.

the neuroleptics hinges on the relationship between exteroceptive stimuli (warning signal and shock).

DISCRIMINATED APPROACH

Might it not be possible to demonstrate the characteristic neuroleptic effect in a situation that does not involve shock at all? Experiments by Migler (1975) and by Clody and Carlton (1980) provide just such a demonstration.

The easiest way to understand the logic of these studies is to first consider the details of discriminated avoidance. It is these details that must be duplicated in a situation that does not involve shock. The relevant information is outlined in Table 16–2.

In discriminated avoidance (the top half of the table) the animal has the opportunity to avoid (R-1) during a pre-shock signal (S-1; row A). If it fails to avoid, a second stimulus (shock; S-2) follows and the animal can escape (R-2; row B).

These relationships are also realized in the discriminated approach procedure used by Migler and by Clody and Carlton (the bottom half of the table). In this case, a signal (S-1) indicates that food reinforcement is available, and a response (R-1) results in the delivery of that reinforcement. However, if the animal fails to emit R-1, reinforcement is still delivered. The sound of the mechanism that delivers reinforcement (S-2) thus provides a signal that food is available and can be claimed (R-2). (These R-2 responses were, in fact, entries into a small well that contained the delivered food pellet.)

Table 16–2

	Stimuli	Response
	Discriminated avoidance	
A.	S-1 (warning signal)	R-1 (avoidance)
B.	S-2 (shock follows R-1 failure)	R-2 (escape)
	Discriminated approach	
C.	S-1 (reinforcement available)	R-1 (delivers reinforcement)
D.	S-2 (reinforcement follows R-1 failure)	R-2 (claim reinforcement)

This procedure differs from most techniques involving positive reinforcement in that the reinforcement is delivered *even if* the animal fails to respond. Thus, R-1 is analogous to avoidance, and R-2, to escape. If this analogy holds, R-1 should be more sensitive to neuroleptic than is R-2, just as avoidance responding is more sensitive than escape responding. That this is the case is illustrated in Figure 16–1.

In the study by Clody and Carlton (1980), the expected differential was obtained with various doses of chlorpromazine. Note, for example, that there was a 63% inhibition of R-1 at 3.0 mg/kg but only a 15% inhibition of R-2 at this same dose. Clody and Carlton also showed that increasing the magnitude of food reinforcement reduced this differential effect on R-1 and R-2. Analogously, increasing the intensity of shock has been shown to decrease the differential effects of neuroleptics on avoidance versus escape behaviors (see Bignami, 1978).

There is, then, a parallel between discriminated avoidance and discriminated approach that confirms our previous idea about exteroceptive stimuli. That is, the selective sensitivity of discriminated avoidance apparently does not lie in the use of shock or avoidance contingencies per se (see Leander, 1981). We will consider that idea again, but let us first examine several other features of the neuroleptic response.[1]

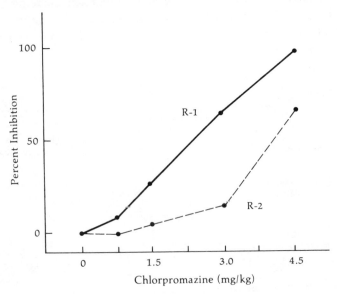

Figure 16–1. Dose–response functions for the effects of chlorpromazine on two response indices (*R-1* and *R-2;* see text). (Data redrawn from Clody, D. E., and Carlton, P. L.: Stimulus efficacy, chlorpromazine, and schizophrenia. *Psychopharmacology* 69:127–131, 1980.)

SECONDARY CLINICAL EFFECTS

Two secondary neuroleptic effects have clear behavioral consequences; these effects are sedation and EPS. What role, if any, do they have in controlling the selectivity seen in our model?

SEDATION

Many of the neuroleptics do produce sedation, but this effect certainly cannot account for the symptom remission they produce. If this were true, then the benzodiazepines, barbiturates, antidepressants, and a host of other drugs would all have clinical efficacy. They do not have such efficacy, and they do not have selective effects in our model.

EPS

As noted in Chapter 13, certain motor effects are collectively called the extrapyramidal syndrome, or EPS, because they are similar to symptoms seen with known dysfunctions in the extrapyramidal system of the brain. EPS may include motor restlessness, rigidity, and tremor similar to that seen in Parkinson's disease, as well as muscle spasms, loss of muscle tone and several other symptoms. These side-effects occur in 40–50% of patients treated with neuroleptics. Fortunately, EPS can be controlled by adjunctive medication. (We will, for simplicity, refer to the several medications that can control EPS as "anti-EPS drugs.")

The relation of EPS and the management of schizophrenic behaviors has two characteristics that are pertinent here. First, anti-EPS drugs are generally very successful in eliminating EPS but do *not* reduce clinical efficacy (see Berger, Elliott, and Barchas, 1978; Klein, Gittleman, Quitkin, and Rifkin, 1980). Second, EPS appears to undergo clinical tolerance despite continued neuroleptic medication. This conclusion is based on the fact that in patients who do initially develop EPS and are given anti-EPS drugs, the latter can often be withdrawn without a reappearance of the extrapyramidal symptoms; EPS does not recur despite the continuation of neuroleptic treatment (see Davis and Cole, 1975). Thus, patients who do develop EPS early in their treatment with neuroleptics may develop tolerance to this initial effect. In contrast, tolerance to beneficial effects is not seen; the control of schizophrenic behaviors achieved by the neuroleptics persists with continued neuroleptic treatment.[2]

Two other facts are relevant here:

1. The anti-EPS drugs are anticholinergic.
2. Cholinomimetics can exacerbate EPS (see Klawans, 1973).

The actions of the cholinomimetics are opposite to those of the anticholinergics, and their reciprocal effects on EPS thus make perfect pharmacologic sense.

Let us now return to our model. We have already seen that the cholinomimetics can mimic the effects of the neuroleptics, and that the anticholinergics can antagonize the effects of the neuroleptics on discriminated avoidance. These facts raise the suspicion that the selectivity seen in our model is closely linked to EPS. Consider Table 16–3. We know that the cholinomimetics have a positive effect on EPS and that they can selectively disrupt discriminated avoidance (row A in the table). We also know that the neuroleptics can induce EPS and that they also have a selective effect on discriminated avoidance (row B). Furthermore, measurement of the effect of the neuroleptics in terms of either EPS or avoidance decrement will show that both are antagonized by anticholinergics (row C). The only factor that does not fit into this parallel pattern is tolerance (row D). Unfortunately, the data pertinent to tolerance are not definitive with respect to either EPS or discriminated avoidance (hence the question marks in row D). It is equally unfortunate that the effect of anticholinergic-plus-neuroleptic has not been studied on a chronic basis in our model.

The latter shortcoming could be a critical one in unraveling the possible relationship of EPS to the discriminated avoidance deficits due to neuroleptic. There is no doubt that anticholinergics do reduce EPS and that they do not antagonize the symptom control achieved with chronic neuroleptic treatment. Thus, the nature of the anticholinergic interaction with *chronic* neuroleptic treatment could prove to be crucial in more securely linking our model to symptom reduction. Unhappily, such data are not available. There is, however, another feature of the neuroleptics

Table 16–3

		EPS	Discriminated avoidance
A.	Cholinomimetics	+	+
B.	Neuroleptics	+	+
C.	Anticholinergics + neuroleptics	−	−
D.	Tolerance	Yes (?)	No (?)

that is pertinent here: different neuroleptics differ in their EPS liability. Clozapine, for example, has a low liability, whereas haloperidol is very likely to produce EPS; chlorpromazine and thioridazine have intermediate liabilities, as shown in Table 16–4. There is a clear parallelism in these data. A drug with low EPS liability (clozapine) has a low potency in our model, and increasing liability is correlated with increasing potency. Now consider the clinical potencies of these drugs.

Different neuroleptics differ in their potencies. Furthermore, the clinical potencies of different neuroleptics are positively correlated with their EPS liability, as illustrated in Table 16–4. That is, as a general rule, the more potent the neuroleptic, the more likely it is to produce EPS. This could mean that the potency correlations we have already considered (see Figure 13–4) are due not to a direct relationship of clinical and laboratory response but to the relationship of potency and EPS. If potency in producing symptom control correlates well with EPS liability, and if EPS liability correlates well with our laboratory response, the clinical and laboratory drug responses will also be strongly correlated. But this correlation could be due to the intervening relations with EPS. In its extreme form, this conclusion suggests that our model is related to clinical drug response only because of a linkage to EPS.

Table 16–5 summarizes these relationships in the context of the various criteria we have used in evaluating discriminated avoidance as a model of the clinical neuroleptic response. The clinical data are summarized in the middle column, and the relations of these data to the model are given at the right.

As far as criterion A is concerned, the clinical data pertinent to the neuroleptics indicate that this criterion could be met because the model shares factors with symptom reduction (efficacy) or with EPS (entry 1 in the table). That is, discriminated avoidance would discriminate neuroleptics from nonneuroleptics if it were sensitive to factors deter-

Table 16–4

EPS liability	Drug	MED in discriminated avoidance*	Average daily clinical dose**
Very low	Clozapine	7.20	1538
Low	Thioridazine	5.00	788
Moderate	Chlorpromazine	1.80	750
High	Haloperidol	0.16	8

*In mg/kg; see Table 13–4.
**In mg; see Table 13–1.

Table 16–5

Criterion	Clinical data	Conclude that model is:
A	Neuroleptics manage symptoms and produce EPS	1. Linked to efficacy or EPS
	Cholinomimetics do not manage symptoms but do exacerbate EPS	2. Linked to EPS
B	Greater neuroleptic potency in symptom management correlated with EPS liability	3. Linked to efficacy or EPS
C	Clinical neuroleptic response delayed	4. Not linked to efficacy
	Tolerance to clinical response does not occur but tolerance to EPS probable	5. Probably linked to efficacy
D	Clinical neuroleptic response not antagonized by anti-EPS medication	6. Probably linked to EPS

mining symptom reduction *or* if it were sensitive to factors determining EPS. These data are thus not definitive. However, the fact that the cholinomimetics exacerbate EPS, do not manage symptoms, but do have specific effects on discriminated avoidance suggests that avoidance is more closely associated with EPS than with symptom management (entry 2). Furthermore, the correlation of clinical potencies and laboratory potencies (criterion B) could be due to a communality between discriminated avoidance and EPS or symptom reduction (entry 3). Again, the data are not definitive.

Criterion C involves two temporal relationships. First, the clinical neuroleptic response is delayed (1 to 3 weeks), whereas the laboratory response is almost immediate; this result suggests that discriminated avoidance behavior is not linked to symptom management (entry 4). Second, tolerance to the clinical response (symptom management) does not develop, whereas our data indicate that tolerance to EPS does, this clinical discrimination of symptom reduction and EPS is paralleled by the meager data available concerning the lack of tolerance of the effects of chronic neuroleptic treatment on discriminated avoidance (entry 5).

Finally, let us consider criterion D. Clinical symptom management due to the neuroleptics is not antagonized by concurrent anti-EPS medication. On the other hand, anticholinergics do antagonize the effects of the neuroleptics on discriminated avoidance, and anti-EPS medications are anticholinergic. We can, therefore, conclude that there is a probable linkage of discriminated avoidance to those processes that control EPS (entry 6).

The data in Table 16–5 certainly do not permit a compelling conclusion about the relation of our proposed model to symptom reduction. Indeed, of the six entries, two (entries 1 and 3) are not definitive, two (entries 2 and 6) favor a linkage to EPS, and one (entry 4) indicates that symptom reduction can be *dis*sociated from the effects of the neuroleptics on discriminated avoidance. Only one item (entry 5) indicates that the model is linked to symptom reduction, but this linkage must be classed as "probable" at best.

This outcome brings us back to an issue we have encountered several times before. With the exception of the data pertinent to tolerance, the laboratory studies we are considering all involve acute medication; in contrast, the clinical data are based on chronic medication. Thus, in order to bring our criteria into contact with clinical reality, we need studies of the effects of chronic neuroleptic treatment on discriminated avoidance. Might tolerance to the effects of the cholinomimetics develop, thus eliminating the conceptual linkage to EPS? Might the effects of chronic neuroleptics not be antagonized by anticholinergics, thus eliminating a second linkage to EPS? We do not yet know the answers to these and other questions.

INTERPRETING THE MODEL

This chapter began with a consideration of the role exteroceptive stimuli may have in controlling the behavior seen in our model. It is tempting to speculate on this idea because a very large literature suggests that deficits in "stimulus processing" characterize schizophrenic disorders. Thus, there may be a relationship between these deficits and the dependence of our model on particular stimulus relationships. (See Clody and Carlton (1980) for a discussion of this prospect and the data pertinent to it.) Such speculation, however, is not truly warranted in the face of the data just considered. In fact, we might just as reasonably speculate on deficits in motor function and movement initiation.

These concerns bring us to the overriding point to be made on the basis of the data we have been considering. We emerged from Chapter 13 with what appeared to be a moderately satisfactory model. It would, therefore, have been easy to concoct a variety of theories about the relationship of this model to schizophrenic behavior. But, when we go through the rather tedious routine of actually analyzing the model in detail, we find that all is not what it at first seemed to be. The fact of the matter is that we do not know if we have a truly satisfactory model because, as we have just seen, we do not have the data necessary to dissociate it from those factors that, first, do control EPS but, second, do not control symptom reduction.

NOTES

1. The traditional interpretation of avoidance responding is that it is maintained because it reduces some internal state of "fear" or "anxiety." In this view, neuroleptics selectively reduce this anxiety and therefore reduce avoidance responding. The data shown in Figure 16–1 make this interpretation suspect. If there is no shock, why should there be any anxiety to be reduced? Furthermore, punishment procedures involve shock and presumed anxiety but are not selectively sensitive to the neuroleptics, as we have seen. (There is also little evidence that the neuroleptics reduce clinical reports of anxiety, as we saw in Chapter 13.) In addition, the anxiolytics do not have selective effects in avoidance procedures. How, then, is it possible for different procedures that all involve shock to be differentially sensitive to different drugs when all engender a presumed state of fear or anxiety? Obviously, the traditional interpretation makes no pharmacologic sense.

   These considerations are also pertinent to the common use of the term "major tranquilizers" to refer to the neuroleptics and of "minor tranquilizers" to refer to the anxiolytics. "Tranquility" implies the absence of anxiety, but neuroleptics clearly do not produce tranquility in this sense. Moreover, the "major–minor" usage implies that neuroleptics and anxiolytics lie on a common pharmacologic dimension, a concept that is patently absurd in light of the available data.

   All in all, interpretations based on presumed states of fear and anxiety, as well as the attendant "major–minor" usage, add up to a severely misguided set of assumptions that are unsupported by fact.

2. The prospect that patients with EPS develop tolerance is inferential. That is, there are no definitive studies of patients given neuroleptics but not given anti-EPS medication. Thus, the course of tolerance to EPS has not been directly monitored. The reason is obvious: to permit the occurrence of EPS and also to withhold efficacious treatment for it would be blatantly unethical.

Chapter 17
Physiologic Mechanisms

IN THIS CHAPTER, we will consider some of the ways in which models can be used to elucidate physiologic mechanism. Because our emphasis will be on the process of analysis itself, we will not consider all of the physiologic mechanisms that have been proposed to account for the actions of the anxiolytics and neuroleptics. Rather, we will focus on two issues: how models can be used and why they are needed. The neuroleptics provide us with an excellent example of the second issue.

THE NEUROLEPTICS AND BRAIN DOPAMINE

Let us begin by considering yet another aspect of the secondary effects that characterize the neuroleptics. As we have already seen, these secondary effects include the following:

1. Antihistaminic effects
2. Anticholinergic effects
3. Adrenergic blocking actions

The first entry indicates that the neuroleptics produce many of the effects of known antihistamines. One of their effects, then, is to attenuate the activities of a naturally occurring substance, histamine. Similarly, the second entry indicates that the neuroleptics share many of the effects of atropine and scopolamine; they can thus be supposed to attenuate the muscarinic activities of acetylcholine (see Chapter 3).

In the third entry, the term "adrenergic" refers to the collective actions of two other naturally occurring substances, epinephrine and norepinephrine. The entry thus indicates that the neuroleptics share some of the activity of drugs known to block the actions of epinephrine and norepinephrine. For example, these two substances are known to be critical to the maintenance of blood pressure. Reductions in blood pressure (hypotension) are therefore produced by the neuroleptics.

HYPOTHESES ABOUT MECHANISM OF NEUROLEPTIC EFFECT

The secondary effects of the neuroleptics naturally lead to several hypotheses about mechanism. Might it be that the neuroleptics act as they do because they attenuate the actions of histamine, acetylcholine, epinephrine, or norepinephrine?

There are two general reasons why these hypotheses do not have much appeal. First, we immediately recognize that there are other antihistamines, other anticholinergics, and other adrenergic blockers, but that none of these is neuroleptic. Second, there are potency relations among the neuroleptics that cast serious doubt on these ideas.

We know that different neuroleptics have different potencies in producing symptom control. These clinical potencies range from the low for chlorpromazine to the high for haloperidol, for example (see Chapter 13). There are also potency differences relevant to the secondary effects of the neuroleptics.

As a general rule, the greater the clinical potency of a neuroleptic, the *lower* its potency in producing antihistaminic, anticholinergic, and adrenergic blocking effects. Chlorpromazine, for example, is much more likely to produce these effects than is haloperidol.

If antihistaminic, anticholinergic, or adrenergic blocking activities were truly the mechanism underlying symptom control, then chlorpromazine would be more potent than haloperidol. At a more general level, the fact that potency in producing these secondary effects is inversely related to clinical potency provides evidence against the idea that histamine, acetylcholine, epinephrine, or norepinephrine is critically involved in the mechanism of neuroleptic action.[1]

EPS AND NEUROLEPTIC EFFECT

As noted in Chapter 16, the likelihood that a given neuroleptic will produce EPS parallels its clinical potency: Higher clinical potency is associated with greater EPS liability (see Table 16–4). This fact suggests that the pathophysiology of EPS might supply a clue about the mechanism of neuroleptic activity. After all, if the two go hand in hand, might they be due to a common mechanism?

Role of Dopamine in Motor Function   EPS is, as we have seen, a shorthand term for an array of disturbances in motor function. The disorder called Parkinson's disease is characterized by many of these same disturbances. It is also known that (1) Parkinson's disease is due to dysfunction in a particular brain locus, the nigrostriatum; (2) the nigrostriatum is *normally* rich in dopamine, or DA; (3) Parkinson's disease patients have DA deficits in this locus; and (4) the symptoms of Parkinson's disease can be controlled by drugs that increase DA activity. It is thus clear that the mechanism of the disease is a deficit in DA activity in a particular brain locus (see Klawans, 1973).

DA Attenuation and Neuroleptic Effect   The fact that the motor disturbance in Parkinson's disease is DA-dependent naturally leads to an idea about the neuroleptics and DA: Might the neuroleptics block the actions of DA to produce motor dysfunction (EPS)? The data from an enormous range of biochemical experiments indicate that this is indeed the case.

There is no question whatsoever that the neuroleptics block DA activity. Because DA is so critically involved in modulating movement, the fact that the neuroleptics produce movement disorders makes perfect sense. However, attenuation of DA activity by the neuroleptics does not necessarily mean that such reduction is also the mechanism of symptom control. The effect could be no more than another in the long list of effects that the neuroleptics produce. How, then, can DA attenuation be convincingly related to symptom reduction?

DA ATTENUATION AND SYMPTOM CONTROL: DIFFERENTIAL TOLERANCE IN DIFFERENT BRAIN LOCI

One way of determining the relationship between DA attenuation and symptom reduction is to examine an issue that we have come across before. The effects of the neuroleptics on symptom control do not undergo tolerance. The issue, then, is whether DA attenuation due to the neuroleptics is similarly resistant.

It will be easier to describe the data bearing on this issue if we adopt a shorthand. We will label the attenuation of DA activity due to the neuroleptics as NIDA (Neuroleptic-Induced Dopamine Attenuation). Let us now ask whether NIDA undergoes tolerance as a consequence of chronic medication.

NIDA can be estimated by biochemical procedures that involve assays of different parts of the brains of experimental animals. It turns out that NIDA undergoes tolerance in some brain loci (the nigrostriatum) but not in others (limbic and frontal areas).[2]

These data have two particularly significant implications. First, the fact that NIDA undergoes tolerance in nigrostriatal structures agrees perfectly with the indication that EPS also undergoes tolerance. That is, there is every reason to believe that NIDA in these loci is the mechanism underlying EPS. Therefore, tolerance of NIDA would be expected to occur in these same loci, and in fact it does.

The second implication relates to the fact that symptom control, unlike EPS, does not tolerate. This finding suggests that the brain loci in which NIDA tolerance does not occur could provide the key to unraveling the mechanism of neuroleptic action. In order to evaluate this possibility we must, of course, convincingly relate NIDA in these brain areas to clinical symptom control. But NIDA cannot be estimated directly in humans. We are, thus, back to the basic reason why models are needed in the first place: The clinical drug response must somehow be brought into the laboratory so that its biochemical determinants can be analyzed. In this instance, a model of the clinical neuroleptic response is required in order to link DA activity to it. As yet, however, there is no fully satisfactory model. The analysis is thus at a standstill.[3]

OTHER DRUGS THAT ALTER DA ACTIVITY

If it is true that all neuroleptics reduce DA activity, we can ask whether all drugs that reduce DA activity are also neuroleptic. To answer this question, let us focus on two drugs, alpha-methyl dopa, AMD, and alpha-methyl tyrosine, AMT. Both of these drugs can reduce DA activity, and both have been studied in humans. Neither has been found to be effective in controlling the symptoms of schizophrenia (see Meltzer and Stahl, 1976).

This negative effect is not, however, all that damaging to the prospect of a linkage of DA attenuation and symptom control. As noted in earlier discussions of false negatives and positives, "no effect" can merely mean that the study was inadequate. In the case of AMD and AMT, it could very well be that the doses were not sufficiently high or that the dose regimen was not maintained for a sufficient period of time. But there are ethical constraints on increasing dose and regimen; the truly relevant experiments may simply be impossible in humans.

Again, we need a model, and again we are confronted with the absence of one. The kind of research that could evolve from the study of AMD and AMT is, like that relevant to NIDA, at a standstill. And these instances are certainly not the only examples that could be used to make the general point that the analysis of physiologic mechanism in biology inevitably requires a laboratory model. In the case we are considering, the promising prospect that DA is a critical factor in the clinical neuroleptic response will not be adequately evaluated until a satisfactory model is developed.[4]

THE ANXIOLYTICS, BENZODIAZEPINE RECEPTORS, GABA, AND SEROTONIN

As we concluded in Chapter 16, our model of the clinical neuroleptic response is not all that we had hoped it might be. This shortcoming leaves us with the problem of analyzing the possible physiologic mechanisms underlying the neuroleptic response, as we have just seen. On the other hand, our model of the clinical anxiolytic response is a substantially more satisfactory one. It seems likely, therefore, that this model should be more useful in analyzing mechanisms relevant to the anxiolytics. We can begin to test that expectation by examining data relevant to specific receptors in the brain.[5]

THE BENZODIAZEPINE RECEPTOR (BDZ-R)

One of the topics discussed in Chapter 3 related to the fact that there must be specific receptors for certain drugs in the brain. In the case of the anxiolytics, it has been possible to actually isolate a receptor for one group, the benzodiazepines.

The documented presence of such a brain receptor for the benzodiazepines—denoted as BDZ-R—does not guarantee, however, that activity at those particular receptors necessarily underlies the anxiolytic properties of the benzodiazepines. Given this consideration, how can we examine the possibility of a link between anxiolytic activity and activity at a BDZ-R?

We cannot approach this problem by direct analysis in humans because we obviously cannot assay human brains for BDZ-R activity. But we can do so in the rat brain, and there is a laboratory model of anxiolytic activity in this species. Thus, because we have an empirically validated model—and only because we do—we can begin to answer questions that would otherwise be unanswerable. We can do so by a process identical to that by which we have already analyzed the relationship of clinical drug response to laboratory response. In short, how well does activity at the BDZ-R meet the four criteria previously discussed?

THE BDZ-R AND CRITERIA A AND B

Activity at the BDZ-R is indexed in terms of the affinity of different drugs for the receptor.[6] As far as criterion A is concerned, we would expect anxiolytics to have high affinities for the BDZ-R and nonanxiolytics to have low affinities. In other words, to what extent does affinity for the BDZ-R generate false positives and false negatives?

As a general rule, affinity for the BDZ-R generates few false positives, but it certainly does generate false negatives. (Recall that our behavioral model does not.) Barbiturates and propanediols have very low affinities for the BDZ-R, yet they are unquestionably anxiolytics. This fact means that the activity of the anxiolytics, as a group, cannot be linked to a single physiologic factor in terms of the BDZ-R. We must, therefore, restrict ourselves to the benzodiazepines for the moment.

With this restriction in mind, let us now ask about criterion B: If the BDZ-R is a link to anxiolytic activity, the affinities of different drugs would be expected to correlate strongly with their potencies in our model; the higher the affinity, the higher the potency. Sepinwall and Cook (1980a, b) have examined just this issue. Their results are plotted in Figure 17–1.

The figure provides a plot of values of K_is against the antipunishment MEDs for 14 different benzodiazepines. The K_i values are an index of affinity for the BDZ-R and are reciprocal to it; low K_i indicates high affinity, as shown at the bottom of the figure. Thus, the relationship of K_i to affinity is like that of MED to potency (note the potency relation shown at the left of the figure.)

There is certainly a positive relationship of affinity and potency, but the IFE of 25.0% indicates that it is not a powerful one. Furthermore, this value does not differ markedly from that previously reported by Braestrup and Squires (1978). In this study, the IFE was 33.1% ($r = 0.743$). Thus, activity at the BDZ-R is telling us something about the effects of the benzodiazepines in our model, but it is not telling us all that much.[7]

THE BDZ-R AND CRITERIA C AND D

Criterion C refers to the temporal characteristics of drug response, and as we found in Chapter 12, differential tolerance separates antipunishment effects from sedation. Given this, we can ask whether activity at

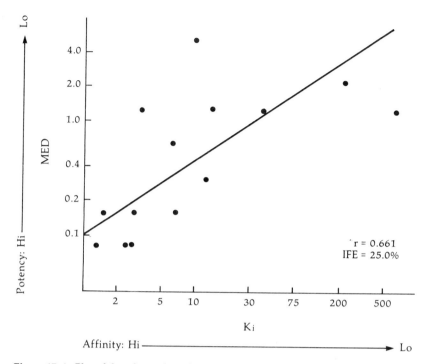

Figure 17–1. Plot of the relationship of K_i (an index of affinity for the BDZ-R) and MEDs in the laboratory model. (Data from Sepinwall, J., and Cook, L.: Mechanism of action of the benzodiazepines: behavioral aspect. *Federation Proceedings* 39:3024–3031, 1980; and from Sepinwall, J., and Cook, L.: Relationship of gamma-aminobutyric acid (GABA) to antianxiety effects of benzodiazepines. *Brain Research Bulletin* 5: 839–848, 1980.)

the BDZ-R is stable in the face of chronic treatment (paralleling the antipunishment effect) or whether there is tolerance (paralleling sedation).

It turns out that the affinity of benzodiazepines for the BDZ-R does not change in response to chronic treatment. This is true for low doses of diazepam (2.0–5.0 mg/kg) given daily for 30 days as well as for extremely high doses (90.0 mg/kg) given daily for 8 weeks. These data provide strong support for the conclusion that activity at the BDZ-R is more closely linked to the anxiolytic effects of the benzodiazepines than to their sedative effects.

Let us now turn to Criterion D and the interaction of the benzodiazepines with other drugs. As noted in Chapter 12, the major clinically relevant interaction is with alcohol, a drug that is active in our model and does potentiate the effect of the benzodiazepines in humans. Alcohol has not, however, been shown to have an affinity for the BDZ-R (Braestrup and Squires, 1978; Vogel and colleagues, 1980). Thus, alcohol can be grouped with the barbiturates and the propanediols; all are anxiolytic but do have have specific activity at the BDZ-R.

OTHER PROPERTIES OF THE BDZ-R

This last fact brings us back to criterion A: The BDZ-R is, at best, an imperfect guide because it is insensitive to several anxiolytics. Furthermore, it is a relatively poor predictor of the potencies of different benzodiazepines in antogonizing the effects of punishment (IFE = 25.0–33.1%).

The properties of the BDZ-R are nonetheless worth examining further because such examination will take us directly into two other important areas. These are, first, the question of whether there is an endogenous anxiolytic in the brain and, second, the linkage of the BDZ-R to gamma-aminobutyric acid (GABA).

Is There an Endogenous Anxiolytic?   When we first encountered the idea of receptors in Chapter 3, it was noted that there must be an endogenous substance that normally acts at the receptor. Thus, the cholinomimetics are drugs that mimic the actions of acetylcholine (ACH) at its receptors; the cholinomimetics can "trick" ACH receptors into responding as if they were occupied by ACH itself. Similarly, if there is an endogenous anxiolytic—EA—analogous to ACH, the benzodiazepines can be thought of as being analogous to the cholinomimetics; the benzodiazepines can "trick" receptors that are normally occupied by EA.

There is some evidence relevant to this prospect, derived from studies of different strains of mice. Different strains differ in the degree of their "emotionality." When some strains are placed in an environment to which they have not previously been exposed, they will move about, actively exploring. In contrast, other more "emotional" strains exposed to the same environment appear to cower in one place and do not explore; there is a suppression of behavior due to the "novelty" of environment. When these more emotional animals are compared with the less emotional ones in terms of BDZ-Rs, it is evident that the former strain has *fewer* BDZ-Rs in their brains (Lippa, et. al.,1979).

Suppose for the moment that there is an EA in the brain and that the receptor for this substance can be identified by the high affinity of the benzodiazepines. (We thus label the receptor as a BDZ-R.) This supposition is logically no different from the idea that cholinomimetics occupy receptors that would normally be occupied by ACH. In that instance, we might label the receptor as a cholinimimetic receptor (CM-R) even though the relevant endogenous substance is ACH.

These relationships are schematized at the top of Figure 17–2, in a format like the one discussed in Chapter 3. The two BDZ-Rs can be occupied by either the endogenous anxiolytic, EA, or by a benzodiazepine, BDZ, to produce anxiolytic activity (at the right). If there were a relative deficit in BDZ-Rs, there should be less net anxiolytic activity due to the endogenous substance and, therefore, *greater* "emotionality." This is precisely the result that has been obtained. We should, however, regard this result with some caution. In the first place, greater emotionality could be due to a variety of factors other than number of BDZ-Rs. A relative deficit could be entirely coincidental. In the second place, the greater emotionality seen in some strains has a relation to anxiolytic activity that relies exclusively on face validity. The measure of emotionality is in no sense an empirically validated model. Thus, these data are at best circumstantial evidence for an endogenous substance that acts at the BDZ-R to produce a "natural" anxiolytic response.

Less circumstantial evidence is available from experiments that have studied changes in the BDZ-R due to exposure to a punishment procedure. In such experiments, it was found that exposure to punishment reduced the the binding of diazepam to the receptor. This effect is schematized at the bottom of Figure 17–2. An array of receptors is shown as available prior to exposure to the punishment procedure *(pre)*. Following exposure *(post)*, some of these receptors are occupied by the EA, and therefore there are fewer sites available for the benzodiazepine. Thus, exposure to punishment should reduce binding of benzodiazepines, and in fact it does.

But if there is evidence for an EA, can it be identified? There have been several candidates proposed, one of which is an endogenous substance called glycine.

Glycine has its own indentifiable receptors in the brain. If glycine were the EA, then the affinities of different benzodiazepines for the glycine receptor should correlate with their potencies in our model; this is precisely the same logic used in developing the relationship shown in Figure 17–1 for the BDZ-R. It turns out that, in this case, there is only a very low correlation ($r = 0.319$). This correlation is not reliably different from zero and provides an IFE of only 5.2%.

These and other data make it clear that glycine is not the EA that normally acts at BDZ-Rs.

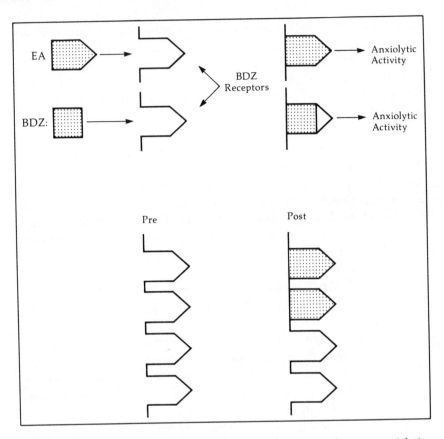

Figure 17–2. Schematic representation of the relationship of an endogenous anxiolytic *(EA)* and a benzodiazepine *(BDZ)* to BDZ-R in producing anxiolytic activity (top); BDZ-Rs before *(pre)* and after *(post)* exposure to punishment procedures (bottom).

The BDZ-R and GABA Another candidate for the EA role is gamma-aminobutyric acid (GABA). GABA is a naturally occurring substance found widely distributed throughout the brain and spinal cord, but unlike most other naturally occurring substances, it is not found in the peripheral nervous system. As a general rule, GABA has an inhibitory function; that is, it reduces neuronal activity. Furthermore, it is clear that, first, the benzodiazepines facilitate the actions of GABA and that, second, GABA is involved in mediating the sedative, muscle relaxant, and anticonvulsant properties of the benzodiazepines. (See Haefely, 1978; Schallek, Horst, and Schlosser, 1979; Schallek and Schlosser, 1979; and the FASEB volume cited in Note 5.)

An elaboration on the experimental bases of these conclusions would take us too far afield. Here we will focus only on the possible relation of GABA activity and anxiolytic activity. Our first question is an obvious one: Is GABA the EA we have been discussing? The answer is that it is not.

If GABA were the EA we are seeking, it would have, of course, a very high affinity for the BDZ-R. But it has essentially no affinity for it. On the other hand, we do know that there are isolable GABA receptors in the brain (GABA-Rs in *A,* at the left of Figure 17–3); furthermore, the activity of GABA at these is facilitated by the activity of benzodiazepines at their receptors (*B,* at the right of the figure).

One implication of the figure is that benzodiazepines with higher affinities for the BDZ-R should show greater facilitation of GABA and, therefore, have greater muscle relaxant, anticonvulsant, and sedative activity. This is indeed the case (see Lippa and colleagues, 1979; Paul, Morganos, Goodwin, and Skolnick, 1980). But our interest is in the relationship of the BDZ-R to GABA as it may bear on anxiolytic activity in our model.

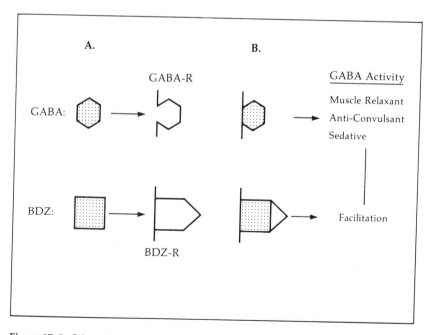

Figure 17–3. Schematic representation of the facilitation of GABA activity at its receptor *(GABA-R)* by the activity of a BDZ at its receptor *(BDZ-R).*

If GABA is involved in mediating the anxiolytic activity of the benzodiazepines, then changes in GABA activity should affect our model in particular ways. In general, the benzodiazepines and GABA work in concert. Thus, decreased GABA activity should have effects opposite to those of the benzodiazepines. On the other hand, increased GABA activity should produce the same effects as those of the benzodiazepines. These expected effects are shown in the left-hand column of Table 17–1. There are several drugs that will either decrease or increase GABA activity; these are listed in the middle column of the table (AOAA is aminooxyacetic acid; 4,5,6,7-tetrahydroisoxazole (5,4-c) pyridin-3-ol is, happily, called simply THIP). The drugs that decrease GABA activity should increase, rather than decrease, suppression. They should also antagonize the benzodiazepines when the drugs are given together (e.g., picrotoxin plus diazepam should produce less of an effect than diazepam alone). The opposite array of effects is to be expected when GABA activity is increased.[8]

The actual results of different experiments designed to evaluate these various interactions are summarized in the third column of the table. Of the 14 studies, only six provide evidence for the possibility that GABA is involved in the mediation of the anxiolytic effects of the benzodiazepines. Clearly, definitive conclusions are not possible, for several reasons.

Table 17–1

Expected effects	Drug	Experimental Results* (+ = agreement with expected effect; − = expected effects not obtained)
Decreased GABA activity Suppression increased; benzodiazepines antagonized	Picrotoxin Bicuculline Thiosemicarbazide	+ + − − + +
Increased GABA activity Suppression decreased; benzodiazepines synergized	AOAA Muscimol THIP Valproic acid	− − + ** − − − − +

*Data adapted from Sepinwall, J., and Cook, L.: Mechanism of action of the diazepines: behavioral aspect. *Federation Proceedings* 39: 3024–3031, 1980; for valproic acid, from Lal, H., Shearman, G. T., Fielding, S., Dunn, R., et al.: Evidence that GABA mechanisms mediate the anxiolytic action of benzodiazepines: a study with valproic acid. *Neuropharmacology* 19: 785–789, 1980.
**Intracerebral injection.

The first reason has to do with the prospect that some of the drugs that are presumed to increase GABA activity may not actually do so in the brain (see Lal and colleagues, 1980). It may be, for example, that muscimol penetrates poorly into the brain following systemic injections. This possibility would account for the negative results itemized in Table 17–1 and would, of course, account for the positive result obtained with intracerebral injections.

A second possibility relates to a phenomenon we have encountered several times before: the differential effects of chronic verus acute treatments. We know that chronic treatment with benzodiazepines provides a differentiation of sedative and anxiolytic effects (see Chapter 12). Unfortunately, it is not yet known whether chronic treatment with the drugs itemized in the table would provide a clarification of the relation of benzodiazepine activity to GABA activity.

A third possibility is also related to an issue we have encountered a number of times before: we have repeatedly seen that the details of procedure can powerfully determine behavioral outcome. The point is a cogent one here because the procedures involved in the studies we are considering have not uniformly incorporated our model. Because procedural detail can so importantly determine experimental result, it is obvious that the use of different procedures could give rise to diverse findings. It is currently impossible to determine the extent to which procedural diversity affects the contradictory results summarized in the table.

Finally, we must consider the possibility that there is more than one BDZ-R. Klepner and coworkers (1979) have provided data indicating that there are at least two BDZ-Rs; one of these is linked to GABA (as in Figure 17–3) but the other is not. There is, thus, the possibility that one BDZ-R is linked to GABA and mediates sedative, anticonvulsant, and muscle relaxant activities, and that another BRZ-R is not linked to GABA and mediates anxiolytic activity. Whether or not this prospect will hold up in the face of further analysis remains to be seen.

OTHER DRUGS WITH ANXIOLYTIC EFFECT: THE BARBITURATES, PROPANEDIOLS, AND ALCOHOL

Barbiturates, propanediol, and alcohol comprise a group of drugs that are anxiolytic but, as we have seen, have no clear relationship to the BDZ-R. However, the actions of the barbiturates and alcohol can, in part at least, be linked to GABA (see Haefely, 1978; Schallek and Schlosser, 1979; Reggiani and colleagues, 1980). The biochemical mechanisms that underlie the actions of the propanediols remain pretty much a mystery.

The general lack of information about these drugs is a serious issue because, if we knew more about them, we could surely better elucidate the mechanisms that control the drug effects seen in our model, and then further clarify the bases of both the clinical anxiolytic response and clinical anxiety itself. As things stand, however, emphasis on the benzodiazepines has edged the other anxiolytics into a shadow of benign neglect that they surely do not deserve.

SEROTONIN (5-HT) AND LABORATORY DRUG RESPONSE

We have yet to consider yet another endogenous substance, called serotonin or 5-hydroxytryptamine, abbreviated 5-HT. Interest in the possible role of brain 5-HT in mediating the effects of punishment can be traced to early reports (Robichaud and Sledge, 1969; Geller and Blum, 1970) on the effects of a drug called *para* chlorophenylalanine, abbreviated PCPA. PCPA depletes the brain of 5-HT and has antipunishment effects comparable to those of the anxiolytics. There is thus a suggestion that 5-HT is involved in mediating the suppression due to the effects of punishment: Deplete 5-HT (with PCPA), and less suppression occurs.

But there is an alternative to this possibility: Might the antipunishment property of PCPA be mediated by some action other than its effect on 5-HT? After all, no drug has a single activity. How, then, can we suppose that the effect of this one drug is due to only one of its actions? The question is an important one because it raises an issue that extends far beyond the relationship of PCPA, punishment, and 5-HT.

Suppose that a given drug has five actions; let us call these ABCDE. The effect of this drug could thus be due to any one of the five or to some interaction among them. Now suppose that a second drug has actions ABFGH. If the two drugs have the same effect, it is at least plausible to suppose that the effect is attributable to AB. If yet another drug has actions ACDEF, and this drug had the same effect as the other two, we could then conclude that the effect is due to A.

As we add more and more drugs to our collection, it becomes progressively more likely that the effect is due to a single common factor. Analysis based on a single drug is at best weak; analysis based on a number becomes more persuasive as that number increases. Given this, let us return to PCPA and 5-HT.

PCPA does deplete the brain of 5-HT, but this fact alone does not necessarily mean much, as we have just seen. As it turns out, there are many ways to reduce the activity of 5-HT, each involving a different drug. These drugs and their effect on 5-HT are summarized in Table 17-2 (see Sepinwall and Cook, 1980a). The important thing about this listing is that *all* of the drugs have been reported to have antipunishment effects. It is thus clear that 5-HT is required for the full expression of punishment-induced suppression. Furthermore, there is the obvious implication that 5-HT in the brain is involved in mediating the effects of anxiolytics in humans.

But there is more to the story than this: If decreased 5-HT activity decreases the effect of punishment, we should be able to show that increased 5-HT activity increases the effect of punishment (i.e., increases the degree of suppression). This brings us to another general rule.

We have already seen that, as more drugs are shown to have a common behavioral effect, the more plausible it is to suppose that this effect is due to a shared action. (In the case we have just considered, the common behavioral effect is attenuated suppression, and the shared action is attenuated 5-HT activity.) We should now be able to go one step further and turn the relationship on its head: Increasing activity should have an opposite behavioral effect. There are, then, two rules to consider in the analysis of the mechanism of a drug: First, a number of drugs with a shared action should be shown to have a common behavioral effect. Second, a number of drugs with an opposite action should have an opposite behavioral effect. (Note that these rules apply in Table 17-1.)

It is obvious that interpretations of mechanism based on the effects of one or two drugs can be regarded only as suggestive and certainly

Table 17-2

Effect on 5-HT	Drug
Depletion	PCPA
	alpha-propyldopacetamide
	5, 6-dihydroxytryptamine*
Antagonism	Methysergide
	Cinanserin
	Bromolysergic acid
	Lysergic acid
	Mescaline
	Cyproheptadine

*Given intraventricularly.

not definitive. Regrettably, we do not have to look far in the relevant literature to find such premature interpretations; they should be viewed with caution. But such caution need not be applied in the case of 5-HT and punishment. This is true because, not only has our first rule been met (Table 17–2), but the effects of several other drugs also meet the second rule.

Three different drugs are pertinent here: 5-hydroxytryptophan, alpha-methyl tryptamine and N, N-dimethyl tryptamine. All increase 5-HT activity, and all three have been found to increase punishment-induced suppression. These data, in combination with those in Table 17–2, suggest that 12 different drugs all affect 5-HT, and that all have an effect that agrees with the idea that 5-HT is involved in controlling suppression. The evidence for this conclusion is strong, but it does not fully address our main concern: the physiologic mechanisms involved in the activity of the anxiolytics themselves.[9]

We would expect that, if 5-HT is truly involved in their action, the anxiolytics would reduce 5-HT activity. As far as the benzodiazepines are concerned, there is evidence that precisely such an effect occurs. But there is essentially no information on the barbiturates, the propanediols, or alcohol. We are, therefore, in much the same position that we were in when we considered GABA: There is compelling evidence that both GABA and 5-HT are crucially involved in anxiolytic action, but this evidence has focused on the benzodiazepines to the virtual exclusion of other but equally important anxiolytics.

We do, nonetheless, know that increased GABA activity can reduce the activity of a variety of endogenous substances, 5-HT among them. There is therefore the distinct possibility that anxiolytics increase GABA activity and thereby decrease 5-HT activity to produce their characteristic effects in our model. But it is important to bear two things in mind when considering this 5-HT–GABA interaction: First, increased GABA activity decreases the activity of several other endogenous substances in addition to 5-HT; second, our data are based exclusively on the benzodiazepines, not on all anxiolytics.[10]

EXTENDING THE ANALYSIS TO HUMANS

One of the criteria discussed in the context of model development concerned direct tests of the model in humans. Without such tests, any model will be weak. The same criterion should be applied to the analysis of physiologic mechanism. The following example illustrates how this can be done.

A group of drugs (the sulfonylureas) can be classified as antidiabetic because they are all useful in controlling late-onset clinical diabetes. They thus fall into a category based on their clinical efficacy, just as the anxiolytics do. Furthermore, these drugs all are known to reduce blood sugar and thereby control diabetes. But what is their mechanism of action? The steps pertinent to answering this question are given in Table 17–3. The clinical phenomenon (1 in column A) with which we are concerned is elevated blood sugar (in B). The clinical drug response (2 in A) is reduced blood sugar due to the sulfonylureas. We can proceed to analyze this drug response by developing a model with which we can study a laboratory drug response (3 in A); in this case it could be reduced blood sugar in the laboratory rat.

The availability of the model permits us to analyze the mechanism by which the sulfonylureas act. It turns out that these agents release insulin from pancreatic cells (4 in B). We know this because if insulin-containing pancreatic cells are experimentally destroyed, the drugs do not lower blood sugar.[11]

The final test of the mechanism must be a clinical one (5 in column A). We must evaluate insulin—not the sufonylureas—in humans. If the analytical chain is accurate, then insulin (the postulated mediator of drug action) should reduce blood sugar in humans—and, of course, it does.

The example of the sulfonylureas, although not historically accurate, emphasizes a critical and often neglected step in the process of analysis. What makes the analysis of the sulfonylureas so compelling is that the presumed mediator itself, not the drugs being analyzed, produce the ex-

Table 17–3

	A	B	C
1.	Clinical phenomenon	Elevated blood sugar; other signs	Report of anxiety; other signs
2.	Clinical drug response	Reduced blood sugar	Report of reduced anxiety
3.	Laboratory drug response	Reduced blood sugar	Antipunishment
4.	Physiologic mechanism	Insulin release	GABA, 5-HT; other
5.	Clinical test	Insulin reduces blood sugar (same as 2)	(?)

pected effect (reduced blood sugar occurs in both 2 and 5). Thus, a complete analysis of drug action requires a manipulation of the presumed mechanism that is independent of the drugs being analyzed. If we fail to undertake that final step, we cannot independently confirm the hypothesis.

Now consider the right-hand column of the table. We have already considered the steps (1 through 4) by which we can move from clinical phenomenon to a clinical drug response, from there to the validation of a model, and then to the use of that model in the process of physiologic analysis. But what about step 5, the final confirmation? Clearly, we need to return to step 2 and analyze the effects of drugs other than the anxiolytics that may modify GABA or 5-HT activity.

There are some possibilities immediately available to us. Picrotoxin, for example, is used clinically and antagonizes the actions of GABA (see Table 17–1). This drug should, if our ideas about GABA are correct, produce reports of increased anxiety (the opposite of the effect of the anxiolytics in step 2). Similarly, two other drugs (cyproheptadine and methysergide; see Table 17–2) have been used in humans and presumably attenuate the actions of 5-HT. Thus, if our ideas about 5-HT are valid, we might be able to show that these drugs produce reports of reduced anxiety.

Neither of these kinds of experiments in humans has been undertaken. Considering the prospect of undertaking them does, nonetheless, serve to highlight three different and important issues.

First, the analysis of anxiolytic activity will not be complete until experiments of the kind discussed here have been completed. More to the point, no analysis of any drug class will be complete until the analysis is extended to humans; laboratory models are powerful tools that can focus attention on isolated factors, but they are not—and can never be—a substitute for coming full circle to the clinic.

The second issue has to do with the prospect that the kinds of experiments we are considering may not work, for two reasons: First, the range of doses that can be studied in humans may be severely limited by the side-effects of these drugs. Second, self-report may be too unreliable a measure for analytical purposes; it may therefore be necessary to rely on the more objective indices discussed at the end of Chapter 12. But even these may not prove to be sufficiently sensitive. Thus, we may come up empty-handed on two counts. It is important to recognize, however, that such a negative outcome would not necessarily invalidate our analysis. It could indicate only that we have yet to develop adequate analytical techniques (recall the earlier discussions of false positives and negatives). A positive result, on the other hand, would go a long way toward validating our analysis. Looked at in this way, there is a great deal to gain and not much to lose.

The third issue takes us back to step 2 in Table 17–3 and a consideration of the clinical drug response itself. Recall that the anxiolytics produce a spectrum of effects in humans. Therefore, the phenomena seen in studies of methysergide and cyproheptadine, for example, should not be expected to be identical to those seen with the anxiolytics. In fact, differences between the spectrum of experimental response and the spectrum of clinical anxiolytic response could provide a way of dissecting the relationship of different behaviors and different physiologic mechanisms. We will return to this idea in the next chapter.

NOTES

1. If one or several of these substances were involved in schizophrenia, then it should be possible to show that schizophrenics are characterized by increases in the activity of the substances in question.
2. Details of the relevant studies can be found in articles by Bacopoulus, Bustos, and Redmond (1978), Bacopoulus, Redmond, and Baulu (1980), and Bacopoulus and colleagues (1979). Excellent reviews of the very large literature on possible biochemical-anatomic substrates in schizophrenia can be found in reports by Meltzer and Stahl (1976), van Kammen (1979), Berger, Elliot, and Barchas (1978), Carlsson (1978), Wyatt (1976), Creese, Burt, and Snyder (1978), and Moore and Kelly (1978).
3. High doses of amphetamine can induce patterns of apparently compulsive grooming, gnawing, and repetitive responding that have been labeled as "stereotypy." Such stereotypy (drug-induced) can be antagonized by the neuroleptics, and the potency of different neuroleptics in doing so correlates well with the clinical potencies of these same drugs (criterion B; see Creese, Burt, and Snyder, 1976). However, (1) cholinomimetics can also induce stereotypy; (2) chronic neuroleptic treatment leads to tolerance of the neuroleptics' antagonism of sterotypy; (3) anticholinergics antagonize the effects of the neuroleptics on stereotypy; and (4) stereotypy itself seems to be mediated by nigrostriatal structures in the brain (see Randrup and Munkvad, 1967; Berger, Elliott, and Barchas, 1978; and Muller and Seeman, 1978). Taken together, these findings indicate that

neuroleptic antagonism of stereotypy is closely linked to EPS and would provide a poor model of the clinical neuroleptic response. Furthermore, it seems that the interaction of the neuroleptics and amphetamine cannot be unequivocally linked to brain DA (see Hornykiewicz, 1978).

4. The lack of an adequate laboratory model has certainly not inhibited the flow of speculation about the physiologic mechanisms that may be involved in schizophrenia. Such speculations are interesting but, in the absence of a satisfactory means of experimental validation, they will continue to be largely idle.

5. Most of the material covered here can be found in articles by Sepinwall and Cook (1978; 1980a, b). In addition, all of the articles in a FASEB volume (*Federation Proceedings* 39: 2943–3056, 1980) should be consulted; they provide a uniformly excellent survey of the status of the field.

6. The affinity of a drug is an indirect index of the extent to which it conforms to a receptor (see Chapter 3).

7. Lippa, Nash, and Greenblatt (1979) have reported somewhat higher values ($r = 0.830$; IFE $= 44.2\%$) with a punishment procedure that is related to our model.

8. In Table 17–1, + entries indicate effects specific to punished behavior. For example, if picrotoxin increased suppression without also producing an overall decrement in responding, that result is indicated by a +. An overall decrement in responding would, of course, increase suppression, but such an effect cannot be taken as a sign of a specific interaction with punishment processes or, by implication, the processes underlying the anxiolytic response.

9. Unfortunately, all of the studies pertinent to 5-HT and punishment have not involved our model. Thus, inferences about 5-HT and the anxiolytic response are somewhat more circumstantial than is desirable.

10. Particularly pertinent here is an elegant study by Wise, Berger, and Stein (1972); also see Stein, Belluzzi, and Wise (1977). Acute benzodiazepine administration was found to decrease the activity of both 5-HT and norepinephrine—NE—in the brain. However, with chronic administration the activity of NE recovered (underwent tolerance), whereas that of 5-HT did not. Stein and his coworkers were also the first to show that the overall depression of responding (indicative of sedation) recovered with chronic treatment, but that the antagonism of punishment-induced suppression (indicative of anx-

iety reduction) did not (see Figure 12–5). Thus, tolerance dissociated two behavioral effects (sedation and punishment antagonism) and two biochemical effects (reduced activities of 5-HT and NE). The nature of this dissociation suggests that 5-HT rather than NE is more critically involved in the anxiolytic response.

11. This means of analyzing the mechanism of action of the sulfony-lureas again emphasizes the importance of laboratory models. Obviously, pancreatic cells could not have been experimentally destroyed in human subjects.

Chapter 18

Physiologic Mechanism, Behavioral Models and the Limits of Analysis

WE BEGAN OUR tour of behavioral pharmacology with a consideration of the ways in which the behavioral effects of drugs can be measured (Chapters 2 and 3). In that context, we soon encountered a note of complexity in the form of rate-dependency (Chapter 4); that note was then amplified by our consideration of drugs as stimuli (Chapters 5, 6 and 7) and of the multiple factors that control tolerance (Chapters 8 and 9). This compounding of complexity then led us to a confrontation with a major question: How is it possible to impose order on the potentially enormous diversity characteristic of the behavioral effects of drugs?

We began to develop an answer to that question by adopting a strategy based on a clinically derived classification (Chapter 10); that strategy dictated, in turn, the need for laboratory models (Chapter 11). Given this need, we then turned to an examination of the question of whether empirically validated models are, in fact, now available to us (Chapters 12, 13 and 14). Further analysis of this question (Chapters 15 and 16) brought us to the final leg of our tour; an examination of the way in which models can be used to elucidate the physiologic mechanisms that underlie drug action (Chapter 17). Thus, in broad outline, we have considered the following:

1. Potential behavioral diversity generates a need for
2. a means of drug classification that is, first, based on behavioral

change (clinical drug responses) and that can, second, be used to validate

3. laboratory models of clinical drug response; these models can, in turn, be used as the basis of

4. analyses of the physiologic mechanisms that underlie clinical drug response itself.

This sequence leads directly to three issues that we have not yet explicitly examined; we will consider these three in the remainder of this Chapter.

ACCOUNTING FOR CLINICAL DRUG RESPONSES

Suppose we were able to isolate a physiologic mechanism involved in the action of a group of drugs. It seems very likely, for example, that an endogenous anxiolytic (EA) that is mimicked by the benzodiazepines will ultimately be found; suppose, then, that an EA, the endogenous substance naturally active at the BDZ-R, has been identified (see Chapter 17). Would that identification lead us to a full account of the clinical anxiolytic response?

It is important to bear in mind that the clinical drug responses with which we have been concerned (e.g., reports of reduced anxiety) are, in fact, changes in behavior. Furthermore, if there is one lesson to be learned from this book, it is that behavioral changes due to drug can only be understood in terms of a complexly interacting system of variables in which drug action itself is only one part; as we have repeatedly seen, behavioral change due to drug cannot be completely understood when it is divorced from either the environmental context or the historical antecedents of the behavior in question. More to the point, manipulations of physiologic mechanism are not fundamentally different from those involved in drug administration. That is, there is no reason whatsoever for supposing that the behavioral changes induced by physiologic manipulations will be immune to interactions within a network of behavioral determinants. Thus, although isolation of a physiologic mechanism may account for a major fraction of behavioral change, it will not automatically lead to a complete account of that change. A simple example, again based on the effects of the sulfonylureas (see Table 17-3), will illustrate the point.

The sulfonylureas are, as we have seen, useful in the management of the symptoms of late-onset diabetes; they thus produce a characteristic clinical drug response. We have also seen that the physiologic mechanism underlying this action is the release of insulin. But this isolation of mechanism cannot fully account for the clinical drug response to either the sulfonylureas or to insulin itself; it cannot do so because symptom control in the diabetic patient (the clinical drug response) cannot be fully understood in the absence of a consideration of other variables that interact with pharmacologic effect (e.g., life stresses, type of diet, carrying out the behaviors involved in self-administration of the prescribed treatment). In the case of the still more complex interactions involved in the behavioral changes we have been considering, the account provided by physiologic mechanism alone can be expected to be still more incomplete.

This is not to say, of course, that identification of mechanism does not represent an enormous advance in understanding; it is to say, however, that an account of a clinical drug response in terms of physiologic mechanism has its intrinsic limits. The latter point is an important one because there is a prevalent belief that the isolation of a single physiologic mechanism will utterly eradicate the complexities involved in the analysis of behavioral change. That belief is wholly unwarranted.

ACCOUNTING FOR CLINICAL PHENOMENA

An analysis of a clinical drug response can form the basis of an analysis of the clinical phenomenon corresponding to that clinical drug response. The logic of this approach has three aspects:

1. Because certain drugs can modify a clinical phenomenon (the clinical drug response),
2. the mechanism of this clinical drug response could
3. elucidate the mechanism underlying the clinical phenomenon itself.

The sulfonylureas can be used to illustrate the point once more.

Suppose we were confronted with a set of symptoms that we label as diabetes (the clinical phenomenon). Also, suppose that we knew that certain drugs (the sulfonylureas) antidoted some of these symptoms (the clinical drug response) but that we did not know the mechanism of action of these drugs. Given this state of affairs, we might undertake an analysis like the one we discussed in Chapter 17 and discover that the mechanism of action of the sulfonylureas is the insulin release that they produce. We could then take the next step and conjecture that a causative factor in diabetes itself is a deficit in insulin; subsequent analysis would prove that conjecture to be correct.

Related assumptions have been involved in attempts to analyze the clinical phenomena with which we have been concerned. Thus, it has been supposed that, if we knew the mechanisms involved in neuroleptic action, we could account for schizophrenia (because the neuroleptics block DA activity, might it not be that an *excess* of DA is involved in schizophrenia?); if we could clarify the mechanism of benzodiazepine action, we could isolate the mechanisms controlling clinical anxiety (if we knew that benzodiazepines mimicked an EA, might it not be that anxious patients are characterized by a *deficit* in EA activity?). These questions involve an entirely plausible set of suppositions. Furthermore, it is certain that analyses of this kind will ultimately prove to be of profound significance in our understanding of anxiety, schizophrenia, mania and depression. Such analyses will not, however, be without their inherent limitations.

The basis of these limitations lies in two facts. First, analyses of the clinical phenomena we have been discussing are linked to clinical drug responses; second, the clinical phenomena are themselves behavioral. As far as the first point is concerned, it is important to recall that the relation of clinical phenomena to their corresponding clinical drug responses is imperfect; not all signs characteristic of the phenomena are antidoted by drug. Accordingly, analyses of clinical phenomena derived from their corresponding clinical drug responses will necessarily be incomplete. Furthermore, to the extent that the analysis of these clinical drug responses rely on laboratory models, the mechanisms derived from the models will be still more remote from the corresponding phenomena. That is, there is a chain of progressive remoteness involved in the steps we considered at the beginning of this Chapter: Clinical phenomena are incompletely represented in clinical drug responses and these are, in turn, incompletely represented in laboratory models (see Table 15-1).

These considerations bring us to the second point: The fact that clinical phenomena are themselves behavioral. Because they are behavioral, clinical phenomena—like clinical drug responses—can be fully understood only in terms of a complexly interacting system in which physiologic mechanism is but one component; a complete account of them can never rest solely on such mechanisms. These clinical phenomena—like any behavior—are not exempt from control by the interactions within the system of variables relevant to them.

This issue is an important one because it also bears on the prevalent idea that physiologic mechanism is the be-all and end-all of analysis, that such mechanisms will provide "magic bullets" that will fully erase behavioral disorders. Although identification of mechanisms will be of enormous ultimate significance, these mechanisms should not be over-valued, should not be expected to fulfill a global explanatory function for which they are intrinsically inadequate.

BIOCHEMICAL AND BEHAVIORAL MODELS

Our discussion of the analysis of physiologic mechanism naturally brings us to another question. Why cannot laboratory models be based on physiologic indices; must these models necessarily be behavioral?

There is, in fact, no reason why biochemical indices could not provide us with satisfactory models of clinical drug responses. For example, if indices of neuroleptic-induced DA attenuation (NIDA) conformed to our criteria, they would then constitute a valuable model of the clinical neuroleptic response. Indeed, if such indices did meet our criteria, we would have very strong evidence supporting the hypothesis that DA is critical to the clinical actions of the neuroleptics and, perhaps, to the etiology of schizophrenia itself. Similarly, the changes in GABA or 5-HT due to anxiolytics could generate validated models of the clinical anxiolytic response. There is, in short, no logical a priori reason why behavioral models should occupy a unique position in the business of model construction.

It seems likely, however, that behavioral models will continue to hold a special, if not unique, position in the process of analysis. This likelihood is also related to the progressive remoteness inherent in the analytical steps that we have previously discussed.

As we have seen, physiologic models are necessarily more remote from the behavioral changes that constitute the clinical drug responses and clinical phenomena to be analyzed. They are, therefore, less likely to be closely related to those clinical processes than are behavioral models. The BDZ-R is a case in point.

There can be no serious doubt that these receptors are critical aspects of the anxiolytic response. Yet the laboratory indices they provide are characterized by false negatives, whereas the behavioral model is not, and they generate a relatively low IFE. Viewed in terms of the progressive remoteness we have already considered, this state of affairs is hardly surprising. That is, when we consider the multiplicity of factors that control anxiety (or schizophrenia, depression, or mania), we must conclude that no one biochemical index is likely to provide us with a fully satisfactory model. On the other hand, clinical phenomena and drug responses are behavioral; it is therefore plausible to suppose that they will be better realized in laboratory indices that are also behavioral.

In this context, it is important to recognize that there is a wealth of biochemical information about each of the drug groups we have discussed: the problem lies not in a shortage of material but in providing ways to make sense out of what is available. It is, for example, one thing to know that neuroleptics attenuate DA; it is quite another to bring that fact into contact with clinical reality.

One of the ways in which such contact has been provided involves a kind of verbal gymnastics. The relevant literature is riddled with speculation that is certainly intriguing but is nonetheless disconnected from the clinical processes to which the neuroleptics pertain. Endless conjecture about the meaning of DA attenuation is possible; there is, however, no analytical tool with which the truly pertinent can be dissected from the merely imaginative. As we have seen, such a dissection will require a satisfactory model of the clinical neuroleptic response.

Similar considerations apply to the antidepressants. It is certainly a scientific gain to know that the antidepressants can, for example, have a variety of well-documented biochemical effects on norepinephrine and 5-HT in brain (see Cooper, Bloom, and Roth, 1978). But this finding alone has no necessary bearing on the clinical efficacy that these drugs have. Again, the juxtaposition of relevant biochemical fact with relevant clinical fact requires a model.

Unfortunately, we have very little understanding of how DA relates to neuroleptic activity or of how norepinephrine and 5-HT may be related to the effects of the antidepressants. In contrast, it is no accident that current understanding of the anxiolytics has begun to form so coherent a picture; we could have simply speculated about the role of glycine, for example, but because we have an empirically validated model, we can quickly cut off the speculation and get on to more important matters.

It is true that one goal of any science is to reduce complexity to progressively simpler terms, as we saw in the transition from diversity to the simplicity of Mendeleev's table and from there to atomic theory. It is also true that analogous transitions about the mechanisms we have discussed will ultimately follow a parallel course. It is not true, however, that such a path will emerge from verbal conjecture that proceeds in the absence of empirical validation. Behavioral models of the kind discussed here can provide for such validation. They are, in effect, bridges between clinical complexity and biochemical simplicity; they are the vital link that permits the evaluation of those hypotheses that are otherwise untestable in humans.

Section 7
Bibliography

Altesman, R., Cole, J. O., and Weingarten, C. H.: Beta-blocking drugs in psychiatry. In Cole, J. O. (ed.): *Psychopharmacology Update.* Lexington MA: Collamore Press, 1980.

Anisman, H.: Aversively motivated behavior as a tool in psychopharmacologic analysis. In Anisman, H., and Bignami, G. (eds.): *Psychopharmacology of Aversively Motivated Behavior.* New York: Plenum Press, 1978.

Anisman, H., Remington, G., and Sklar, L. S. Effect of inescapable shock on subsequent escape performance: catecholaminergic and cholinergic mediation of response initiation and maintenance. *Psychopharmacology* 61: 107–124, 1979.

Bacopoulos, N. G., Bustos, G., and Redmond, D. E.: Regional sensitivity of primate brain dopaminergic neurons to haloperidol: alterations following chronic treatment. *Brain Research* 157: 396–401, 1978.

Bacopoulos, N. G., Redmond, D. E., and Baulu, J.: Chronic haloperidol or fluphenazine: effects on dopamine metabolism in brain, cerebrospinal fluid and plasma of *Cercopithecus aethiops* (vervet monkey). *Journal of Pharmacology and Experimental Therapeutics* 212: 1–5, 1980.

Bacopoulos, N. G., Spokes, E. G., Bird, E. D., et al.: Antipsychotic drug action in schizophrenic patients: effect on cortical dopamine metabolism after long-term treatment. *Science* 205: 1405–1407, 1979.

Balster, R. L., and Woolverton, W. L.: Unlimited access intravenous drug self-administration in rhesus monkeys. *Federation Proceedings* 41: 211–215, 1982.

Barrett, J. E., and Stanley, J. A.: Effects of ethanol on multiple fixed-interval fixed-ratio schedule performances: dynamic interactions at different fixed-ratio values. *Journal of the Experimental Analysis of Behavior* 34: 185–198, 1980.

Beer, B., and Migler, B.: Effects of diazepam on galvanic skin response and conflict in monkeys and humans. In Sudilovsky, A., Gershon, S., and Beer, B. (eds.): *Predictability in Psychopharmacology: Preclinical and Clinical Correlations.* New York: Raven Press, 1975.

Berger, B. C., and Stein, L.: Asymmetrical dissociation of learning between scopolamine and Wy 4036, a new benzodiazepine tranquilizer. *Psychopharmacologia (Berlin)* 14: 351–358, 1969.

Berger, P. A., Elliott, G. R., and Barchas, J. D.: Neuroregulators and schizophrenia. In Lipton, M. A., DiMascio, A., and Killam, K. F. (eds.): *Psychopharmacology: A Generation of Progress.* New York: Raven Press, 1978.

Bignami, G.: Effects of neuroleptics, ethanol, hypnotic-sedatives, tranquilizers, narcotics, and minor stimulants in aversive paradigms. In Anisman, H., and Bignami, G. (eds.): *Psychopharmacology of Aversively Motivated Behavior.* New York: Plenum Press, 1978.

Bignami, G., and Michalek, H.: Cholinergic mechanisms and aversively motivated behaviors. In Anisman, H., and Bignami, G. (eds.), *Psychopharmacology of Aversively Motivated Behavior.* New York: Plenum Press, 1978.

Bowden, C. L., and Giffen, M. B.: *Psychopharmacology for Primary Care Physicians.* Baltimore: Williams & Wilkins, 1978.

Braestrup, C., and Squires, R. F.: Brain specific benzodiazepine receptors. *British Journal of Psychiatry* 133: 249–260, 1978.

Bronowski, J.: *The Ascent of Man.* Boston: Little, Brown, 1973.

Browne, R. G.: Effects of antidepressants and anticholinergics in a mouse "behavioral despair" test. *European Journal of Pharmacology* 58: 331–334, 1979.

Bunney, W. E., Jr.: Psychopharmacology of the switch process in affective illness. In Lipton, M. A., DiMascio, A., and Killam, K. F. (eds.): *Psychopharmacology: A Generation of Progress.* New York: Raven Press, 1978.

Cairncross, K. D., Cox, B., Forster, C., and Wren, A. F.: A new model for the detection of antidepressant drugs: olfactory bulbectomy in the rat compared with existing models. *Journal of Pharmacological Methods* 1: 131–143, 1978.

Campbell, J. C., and Seiden, L. S.: Performance influence on the development of tolerance to amphetamine. *Pharmacology, Biochemistry and Behavior* 1: 703–708, 1973.

Carey, R. J.: Disruption of timing behavior following amphetamine withdrawal. *Physiological Psychology* 1: 9–12, 1973.

Carlsson, A.: Antipsychotic drugs, neurotransmitters, and schizophrenia. *American Journal of Psychiatry* 135: 164–173, 1978.

Carlton, P. L.: Potentiation of the behavioral effects of amphetamine by imipramine. *Psychopharmacologia (Berlin)* 2: 364–376, 1961.

Carlton, P. L.: Cholinergic mechanisms in the control of behavior by the brain. *Psychological Review* 70: 19–39, 1963.

Carlton, P. L., and Didamo, P.: Augmentation of the behavioral effects of amphetamine by atropine. *Journal of Pharmacology and Experimental Therapeutics* 134: 91–96, 1961.

Carlton, P. L., Siegel, J. L., Murphree, H. B., and Cook, L.: Effects of diazepam on operant behavior in man. *Psychopharmacology* 73: 314–317, 1981.

Carlton, P. L., and Wolgin, D. L.: Contingent tolerance to the anorexigenic effects of amphetamine. *Physiology and Behavior* 7: 221–223, 1971.

Chen, C-S.: A study of the alcohol-tolerance effect and an introduction of a new behavioural technique. *Psychopharmacologia (Berlin)* 12: 433–440, 1968.

Clody, D. E., and Beer, B.: Conditioned avoidance: a predictor of efficacy and duration of action for long-acting neuroleptic agents. In Sudilovsky, A., Gershon, S., and Beer, B. (eds.): *Predictability in Psychopharmacology: Preclinical and Clinical Correlations.* New York: Raven Press, 1975.

Clody, D. E., and Carlton, P. L.: Stimulus efficacy, chlorpromazine, and schizophrenia. *Psychopharmacology* 69: 127–131, 1980.

Cook, L., and Catania, A. C.: Effects of drugs on avoidance and escape behavior. *Federation Proceedings* 23: 818–835, 1964.

Cook, L., and Davidson, A. B.: Effects of behaviorally active drugs in a conflict–punishment procedure in rats. In Garattini, S., Mussini, E., and Randall, L. O. (eds.): *The Benzodiazepines.* New York: Raven Press, 1973.

Cook, L., and Sepinwall, J.: Psychopharmacological parameters of emotion. In Levi, L. (ed.): *Emotions—Their Parameters and Measurement.* New York: Raven Press, 1975.

Cook, L., and Sepinwall, J.: Reinforcement schedules and extrapolations to humans from animals in behavioral pharmacology. In Weiss, B., and Laties, V. G. (eds.): *Behavioral Pharmacology: The Current Status.* New York: Plenum Press, 1976.

Cook, L., and Weidley, E.: Behavioral effects of some psychopharmacological agents. *Annals of the New York Academy of Sciences* 66: 740–752, 1957.

Cooper, J. R., Bloom, F. E., and Roth, R. H.: *The Biochemical Basis of Neuropharmacology.* New York: Oxford University Press, 1978.

Corfield-Sumner, P. K., and Stolerman, I. P.: Behavioral tolerance. In Blackman, D. E., and Sanger, D. J. (eds.): *Contemporary Research in Behavioral Pharmacology.* New York: Plenum Press, 1978.

Courvoisier, S., Fournel, J., Ducrot, R., Kolsky, M., et al.: Proprietes pharmacodynamiques du chlorhydrate de chloro-3 (dimethyl-amino-3 propyl)-10 phenothiazine (4560 R.P.). Etude experimentale d'un nouveau corps utilisé dans 1 anesthesie potentialisée et dans 1 hibernation artificielle. *Archives Internationales de Pharmacodynamie et Therapeutique* 92: 305–361, 1953.

Creese, I., Burt, D. R., and Snyder, S. H.: Dopamine receptor binding predicts clinical and pharmacological potencies of antischizophrenic drugs. *Science* 192: 481–483, 1976.

Cronbach, L. J.: *Essentials of Psychological Testing,* 3rd ed. New York: Harper & Row, 1970.

Davidson, A. B., and Weidley, E.: Differential effects of neuroleptic and other psychotropic agents on acquisition of avoidance in rats. *Life Sciences* 18: 1279–1284, 1976.

Davis, J. M., and Cole, J. O.: Antipsychotic drugs. In Freedman, A. M., Kaplan, H. I., and Sadock, B. J. (eds.): *Comprehensive Textbook of Psychiatry/II.* Baltimore: Williams & Wilkins, 1975.

Debus, G., and Janke, W.: Methods and methodological considerations in measuring anti-anxiety effects of tranquilizing drugs. *Progress in Neuro-psychopharmacology* 4: 391–404, 1980.

Deneau, G., Yanagita, T., and Seevers, M. H.: Self-administration of psychoactive substances by the monkey. *Psychopharmacologia (Berlin)* 16: 30–48, 1969.

Dews, P. B.: Studies on behavior. I. Differential sensitivity to pentobarbital of pecking performance in pigeons depending on the schedule of reward. *Journal of Pharmacology and Experimental Therapeutics* 113: 393–401, 1955.

Dews, P. B., and DeWeese, J.: Schedules of reinforcement. In Iversen, L. L., Iversen, S. D., and Snyder, S. H. (eds.): *Handbook of Psychopharmacology*, vol. 7. New York: Plenum Press, 1977.

Dews, P. B., and Wenger, G. R.: Rate-dependency of the behavioral effects of amphetamine. In Thompson, T., and Dews, P. B. (eds.): *Advances in Behavioral Pharmacology*, vol. 1. New York: Academic Press, 1977.

Diagnostic and Statistical Manual of Mental Disorders, 3rd ed. Washington DC: American Psychiatric Association, 1980.

Ferster, C. B., and Skinner, B. F.: *Schedules of Reinforcement.* New York: Appleton-Century-Crofts, 1957.

File, S. E., and Hyde, J. R. G.: A test of anxiety that distinguishes between the actions of benzodiazepines and those of other minor tranquilisers and of stimulants. *Pharmacology, Biochemistry and Behavior* 11: 65–69, 1979.

Fischman, M. W., and Schuster, C. R.: The effects of chlorpromazine and pentobarbital on behavior maintained by electric shock or point loss avoidance in humans. *Psychopharmacology* 66: 3–11, 1979.

Fischman, M. W., Schuster, C. R., and Uhlenhuth, E. H.: Extension of animal models to clinical evaluation of antianxiety agents. In Hanin, I., and Usdin, E. (eds.): *Animal Models in Psychiatry and Neurology.* New York: Pergamon Press, 1977.

Fischman, M. W., Smith, R. C., and Schuster, C. R.: The effects of chlorpromazine on avoidance and escape responding in humans. *Pharmacology, Biochemistry and Behavior* 4: 111–114, 1976.

Geller, I., and Blum, K.: The effect of 5-HTP on para-chlorophenylalanine (p-CPA) attenuation of "conflict" behavior. *European Journal of Pharmacology* 9: 319–324, 1970.

Geller, I., Kulak, J. T., Jr., and Seifter, J.: The effects of chlordiazepoxide and chlorpromazine on a punishment discrimination. *Psychopharmacologia (Berlin)* 3: 374–385, 1962.

Geller, I., and Seifter, J.: The effects of meprobamate, barbiturates, d-amphetamine and promazine on experimentally induced conflict in the rat. *Psychopharmacologia (Berlin)* 1: 482–492, 1960.

Geller, I., and Seifter, J.: The effects of mono-urethans, di-urethans and barbiturates on a punishment discrimination. *Journal of Pharmacology and Experimental Therapeutics* 136: 284–288, 1962.

Gerbino, L., Oleshansky, M., and Gershon, S.: Clinical use and mode of action of lithium. In Lipton, M. A., DiMascio, A., and Killam, K. F. (eds.): *Psychopharmacology: A Generation of Progress.* New York: Raven Press, 1978.

Goldberg, S. R., and Schuster, C. R.: Conditioned suppression by a stimulus associated with nalorphine-dependent monkeys. *Journal of the Experimental Analysis of Behavior* 10: 235–242, 1967.

Griffiths, R. R., Brady, J. V., and Bradford, L. D.: Predicting the abuse liability of drugs with animal drug self-administration procedures: psychomotor stimulants and hallucinogens. In Thompson, T., and Dews, P. B. (eds.): *Advances in Behavioral Pharmacology*, vol. 2. New York: Academic Press, 1979.

Groves, P. M., and Thompson, R. F.: Habituation: a dual-process theory. *Psychological Review* 5: 419–450, 1970.

Guilford, J. P.: *Psychometric Methods.* New York: McGraw-Hill, 1936.

Haefely, W. E.: Central actions of benzodiazepines: general introduction. *British Journal of Psychiatry* 133: 231–238, 1978.

Harrell, E. H., Haynes, J. R., Lambert, P. L., and Sininger, R. A.: Reversal of learned helplessness by peripheral arousal. *Psychological Reports* 43: 1211–1217, 1978.

Heffner, T. G., Drawbaugh, R. B., and Zigmond, M. J.: Amphetamine and operant behavior in rats: relationship between drug effect and control response rate. *Journal of Comparative and Physiological Psychology* 86: 1031–1043, 1974.

Heise, G. A., and Boff, E.: Behavioral determination of time and dose parameters of monoamine oxidase inhibitors. *Journal of Pharmacology and Experimental Therapeutics* 129: 155–162, 1960.

Heise, G. A., and Boff, E.: Continuous avoidance as a base-line for measuring behavioral effects of drugs. *Psychopharmacologia (Berlin)* 3: 264–282, 1962.

Hill, R. T., and Tedeschi, D. H.: Animal testing and screening procedures in evaluating psychotropic drugs. In Rech, R. H., and Moore, K. E. (eds.): *An Introduction to Psychopharmacology.* New York: Raven Press, 1971.

Holtzman, S. G.: Tolerance to the stimulant effects of morphine and pentazocine on avoidance responding in the rat. *Psychopharmacologia (Berlin) 39:* 23–37, 1974.

Honigfeld, G., and Howard, A.: *Psychiatric Drugs,* 2nd ed. New York: Academic Press, 1978.

Hornykiewicz, O.: Psychopharmacological implications of dopamine and dopamine antagonists: a critical evaluation of current evidence. *Neuroscience* 3: 773–783, 1978.

Houser, V. P.: The effects of drugs on behavior controlled by aversive stimuli. In Blackman, D. E., and Sanger, D. J. (eds.): *Contemporary Research in Behavioral Pharmacology.* New York: Plenum Press, 1978.

Huesmann, L. R.: Learned helplessness. *Journal of Abnormal Psychology* 87: 1–198, 1978.

Iversen, S. D.: Animal models of anxiety and benzodiazepine actions. *Arznzneimittel-Forschung* 30: 862–868, 1980.

Jaffe, B.: *Crucibles: The Story of Chemistry.* CT: Fawcett Publications, 1957.

Janke, W.: Psychometric and psychophysiological actions of antipsychotics in men. In Hoffmeister, F., and Stille, G. (eds.): *Handbook of Experimental Pharmacology,* vol. 55/I. New York: Springer-Verlag, 1980.

Johanson, C. E.: Drugs as reinforcers. In Blackman, D. E., and Sanger, D. J. (eds.): *Contemporary Research in Behavioral Pharmacology.* New York: Plenum Press, 1978.

Katz, R. J.: Animal models and human depressive disorders. *Neuroscience and Biobehavioral Reviews* 5: 231–246, 1981.

Kelleher, R. T., and Morse, W. H.: Determinants of the specificity of behavioral effects of drugs. *Ergebnisse der physiologie, Biologischen Chemie und Experimentellen Pharmakologie* 60: 1–56, 1968.

Kessler, K. A.: Tricyclic antidepressants: mode of action and clinical use. In Lipton, M. A., DiMascio, A., and Killam, K. F. (eds.): *Psychopharmacology: A Generation of Progress.* New York: Raven Press, 1978.

Kieffer, W. F.: *Chemistry: A Cultural Approach.* New York: Harper & Row, 1971.

Klawans, H. L.: *The Pharmacology of Extrapyramidal Movement Disorders.* New York: S. Karger, 1973.

Klein, D. F., Gittelman, R., Quitkin, F., and Rifkin, A.: *Diagnosis and Drug Treatment of Psychiatric Disorders: Adults and Children,* 2nd ed. Baltimore: Williams & Wilkins, 1980.

Klepner, C. A., Lippa, A. S., Benson, D. I., Sano, M. C., et al.: Resolution of two biochemically and pharmacologically distinct benzodiazepine receptors. *Pharmacology, Biochemistry and Behavior* 11: 457–462, 1979.

Kornetsky, C.: Animal models: promises and problems. In Hanin, I., and Usdin, E. (eds.): *Animal Models in Psychiatry and Neurology.* New York: Pergamon Press, 1977.

Kornetsky, C., and Bain, G.: Morphine: single-dose tolerance. *Science* 162: 1011–1012, 1968.

Ksir, C.: Rate-convergent effects of drugs. In Thompson, T., Dews, P. B., and McKim, W. A. (eds.): *Advances in Behavioral Pharmacology,* vol. 3. New York: Academic Press, 1981.

Kuribara, H.: Effects of repeated administration of d-amphetamine on Sidman avoidance responding in rats. *Psychopharmacology* 71: 105–107, 1980.

Kuribara, H., and Tadokoro, S.: Study of accumulation of fluphenazine enanthate and fluphenazine decanoate, long-acting neuroleptic drugs, after repeated administrations by means of their inhibitory effects on the discriminated avoidance response in rats. *Journal of Toxicological Sciences* 4: 87–98, 1979.

Laffan, R. J., High, J. P., and Burke, J. C.: The prolonged action of fluphenazine enanthate in oil after depot injection. *International Journal of Neuropsychiatry* 1: 300–306, 1965.

Lal, H., Shearman, G. T., Fielding, S., Dunn, R., et al.: Evidence that GABA mechanisms mediate the anxiolytic action of benzodiazepines: a study with valproic acid. *Neuropharmacology* 19: 785–789, 1980.

Leander, J. D.: Rate-dependence and the effects of phenothiazine antipsychotics in pigeons. In Thompson, T., Dews, P. B., and McKim, W. A. (eds.): *Advances in Behavioral Pharmacology,* vol. 3. New York: Academic Press, 1981.

LeBlanc, A. E., Gibbins, R. J., and Kalant, H.: Behavioral augmentation of tolerance to ethanol in the rat. *Psychopharmacologia (Berlin)* 30: 117–122, 1973.

Leshner, A. I., Remler, H., Biegon, A., and Samuel, D.: Desmethylimipramine (DMI) counteracts learned helplessness in rats. *Psychopharmacology* 66: 207–208, 1979.

Lippa, A. S., Nash, P. A., and Greenblatt, E. N.: Pre-clinical neuropsycho-pharmacological testing procedures for anxiolytic drugs. In Fielding, S., and Lal, H. (eds.): *Anxiolytics.* New York: Futura, 1979.

Ludwig, A. M.: *Principles of Clinical Psychiatry.* New York: Free Press, 1980.

Maffii, G.: The secondary conditioned response of rats and the effects of some psychopharmacological agents. *Journal of Pharmacy and Pharmacology* 11: 129–139, 1959.

Maier, S. F., and Coon, D. J.: Long-term analgesic effects of inescapable shock and learned helplessness. *Science* 206: 91–93, 1979.

Matthysee, S., and Haber, S.: Animal models of schizophrenia. In Ingle, D. J., and Shein, H. M. (eds.): *Model Systems in Biological Psychiatry.* Cambridge MA: MIT Press, 1975.

McGuire, P. S., and Seiden, L. S.: The effects of tricyclic antidepressants on performance under a differential-reinforcement-of-low-rates schedule in rats. *Journal of Pharmacology and Experimental Therapeutics* 214: 635–641, 1980.

McKearney, J. W.: The relative effects of d-amphetamine, imipramine and harmaline on tetrabenazine suppression of schedule-controlled behavior in the rat. *Journal of Pharmacology and Experimental Therapeutics* 159: 429–440, 1968.

McKearney, J. W.: Drug effects and the environmental control of behavior. *Pharmacological Reviews* 27: 429–436, 1976.

McKim, W. A.: Rate-dependency: a nonspecific behavioral effect of drugs. In Thompson, T., Dews, P. B., and McKim, W. A. (eds.): *Advances in Behavioral Pharmacology,* vol. 3. New York: Academic Press, 1981.

Meltzer, H. Y., and Stahl, S. M.: The dopamine hypothesis of schizophrenia: a review. *Schizophrenia Bulletin* 2: 19–76, 1976.

Miczek, K. A.: Effects of scopolamine, amphetamine and benzodiazepines on conditioned suppression. *Pharmacology, Biochemistry and Behavior* 1: 401–411, 1973a.

Miczek, K. A.: Effects of scopolamine, amphetamine and chlordiazepoxide on punishment. *Psychopharmacologia (Berlin)* 28: 373–389, 1973b.

Migler, B.: Conditioned approach: an analogue of conditioned avoidance; effects of chlorpromazine and diazepam. *Pharmacology, Biochemistry and Behavior* 3: 961–965, 1975.

Millenson, J. R., and Leslie, J.: The conditioned emotional response (CER) as a baseline for the study of anti-anxiety drugs. *Neuropharmacology* 13: 1–9, 1974.

Mirsky, A. F., and Kornetsky, C.: The effect of centrally-acting drugs of attention. In Efron, D. H., Cole, J. O., Levine, J., and Wittenborn, J. R. (eds.): *Psychopharmacology: A Review of Progress 1957–1967.* Washington DC: U.S. Government Printing Office, 1968. (Public Health Service Publication No. 1836.)

Moore, K. E., and Kelly, P. H.: Biochemical pharmacology of mesolimbic and mesocortical dopaminergic neurons. In Lipton, M. A., DiMascio, A., and Killam, K. F. (eds.): *Psychopharmacology: A Generation of Progress.* New York: Raven Press, 1978.

Morse, W. H., McKearney, J. W., and Kelleher, R. T.: Control of behavior by noxious stimuli. In Iversen, L. L., Iversen, S. D., and Snyder, S. H. (eds.): *Handbook of Psychopharmacology,* vol. 7. New York: Plenum Press, 1977.

Muller, P., and Seeman, P.: Dopaminergic supersensitivity after neuroleptics: time-course and specificity. *Psychopharmacology* 60: 1–11, 1978.

Norton, S.: The study of sequences of motor behavior. In Iversen, L. L., Iversen, S. D., and Snyder, S. H. (eds.): *Handbook of Psychopharmacology*, vol. 7. New York: Plenum Press, 1977.

Overton, D. A.: State-dependent or "dissociated" learning produced with pentobarbital. *Journal of Comparative and Physiological Psychology* 57: 3–12, 1964.

Overton, D. A.: Experimental methods for the study of state-dependent learning. *Federation Proceedings* 33: 1800–1813, 1974.

Overton, D. A.: Drug state-dependent learning. In Jarvik, M. E. (ed.): *Psychopharmacology in the Practice of Medicine*. New York: Appleton-Century, 1977.

Patel, J. B., Ciofalo, V. B., and Iorio, L. C.: Benzodiazepine blockade of passive-avoidance task in mice: a state-dependent phenomenon. *Psychopharmacology* 61: 25–28, 1979.

Paul, S. M., Marangos, P. J., Goodwin, F. K., and Skolnick, P.: Brain-specific benzodiazepine receptors and putative endogenous benzodiazepine-like compounds. *Biological Psychiatry* 15: 407–428, 1980.

Pfeiffer, C. C., and Jenney, E. H.: The inhibition of the conditioned response and the counteraction of schizophrenia by muscarinic stimulation of the brain. *Annals of The New York Academy of Sciences* 66: 753–764, 1957.

Pickens, R.: Behavioral pharmacology: a brief history. In Thompson, T., and Dews, P. B. (eds.): *Advances in Behavioral Pharmacology*, vol. 1. New York: Academic Press, 1977.

Poling, A., Cleary, J., and Monaghan, M.: The use of human observers in psychopharmacological research. *Pharmacology, Biochemistry and Behavior* 13: 243–246, 1980.

Porsolt, R. D., Bertin, A., and Jalfre, M.: Behavioural despair in mice: a primary screening test for antidepressants. *Archives Internationales de Pharmacodynamie et de Therapie* 229: 327–336, 1977.

Porsolt, R. D., Anton, G., Blavet, N., and Jalfre, M.: Behavioural despair in rats: a new model sensitive to antidepressant treatments. *European Journal of Pharmacology* 47: 379–391, 1978.

Randrup, A., and Munkvad, I.: Stereotyped activities produced by amphetamine in several animal species and man. *Psychopharmacologia (Berlin)* 11: 300–310, 1967.

Rapoport, J. L., Buchsbaum, M. S., Zahn, T. P., Weingartner, H., et al.: Dextroamphetamine: cognitive and behavioral effects in normal prepubertal boys. *Science* 199: 560–563, 1978.

Rawlins, N. N. P., Feldon, J., Salmon, P., Gray, J. A., et al.: The effects of chlordiazepoxide HCl administration upon punishment and conditioned suppression in the rat. *Psychopharmacology* 70: 317–322, 1980.

Reggiani, A., Barbaccia, M. L., Spano, P. F., and Trabucchi, M.: Acute and chronic ethanol administration on specific ^{3}H-GABA binding in different rat brain areas. *Psychopharmacology* 67: 261–264, 1980.

Reynolds, G. S.: *A Primer of Operant Conditioning*. Glenview IL: Scott Foresman, 1968.

Rickels, K., Downing, R. W., and Winokur, A.: Antianxiety drugs: clinical use in psychiatry. In Iversen, L. L., Iversen, S. D., and Snyder, S. H. (eds.): *Handbook of Psychopharmacology*, vol. 13. New York: Plenum Press, 1978.

Robbins, T. W.: A critique of the methods available for the measurement of spontaneous activity. In Iverson, L. L., Iverson, S. D., and Snyder, S. H. (eds.): *Handbook of Psychopharmacology*, vol. 7. New York: Plenum Press, 1977.

Robichaud, R. D., and Sledge, K. L.: The effects of p-chlorophenylalanine on experimentally induced conflict in the rat. *Life Sciences* 8: 965–969, 1969.

Sanger, D. J., and Blackman, D. E.: Rate-dependent effects of drugs: a review of the literature. *Pharmacology, Biochemistry and Behavior* 4: 73–83, 1976.

Sanger, D. J., and Blackman, D. E.: Rate-dependence and the effects of benzodiazepines. In Thompson, T., Dews, P. B., and McKim, W. A. (eds.): *Advances in Behavioral Pharmacology*, vol. 3. New York: Academic Press, 1981.

Sansone, M.: Effects of repeated administration of chlordiazepoxide on spontaneous locomotor activity in mice. *Psychopharmacology* 66: 109–110, 1979.

Schallek, W., Horst, W. D., and Schlosser, W.: Mechanisms of action of benzodiazepines. In Hawking, et al. W., (eds.): *Advances in Pharmacology and Chemotherapy*, vol. 16. New York: Academic Press, 1979.

Schallek, W., and Schlosser, W.: Neuropharmacology of sedatives and anxiolytics. *Modern Problems of Pharmacopsychiatry* 14: 157–173, 1979.

Schechter, M. D., and Chance, W. T.: Non-specificity of "behavioral despair" as an animal model of depression. *European Journal of Pharmacology* 60: 139–142, 1979.

Scheckel, C. L., and Boff, E.: Behavioral effects of interacting imipramine and other drugs with d-amphetamine, cocaine, and tetrabenazine. *Psychopharmacologia (Berlin)* 5: 198–208, 1964.

Schuster, C. R., and Balster, R. L.: The discriminative stimulus properties of drugs. In Thompson, T., and Dews, P. B. (eds.): *Advances in Behavioral Pharmacology*. New York: Academic Press, 1977.

Schuster, C. R., Dockens, W. S., and Woods, J. H.: Behavioral variables affecting the development of amphetamine tolerance. *Psychopharmacologia (Berlin)* 9: 170–82, 1966.

Schuster, C. R., and Johanson, C. E.: An analysis of drug-seeking behavior in animals. *Neuroscience and Biobehavioral Reviews* 5: 315–323, 1981.

Schuster, C. R., Renault, P. F., and Blaine, J.: Analysis of the relationship of psychopathology to non-medical drug use. In Pickens, R. W., and Heston, L. L. (eds.): *Psychiatric Factors in Drug Abuse*. New York: Grune & Stratton, 1979.

Schuster, C. R., and Zimmerman, J.: Timing behavior during prolonged treatment with dl-amphetamine. *Journal of the Experimental Analysis of Behavior* 4: 327–330, 1961.

Seligman, M. E. P.: *Helplessness*. San Francisco: W. H. Freeman, 1975.

Sepinwall, J., and Cook, L.: Behavioral pharmacology of antianxiety drugs. In Iversen, L. L., Iversen, S. D., and Snyder, S. H. (eds.): *Handbook of Psychopharmacology*, vol. 13. New York: Plenum Press, 1978.

Sepinwall, J., and Cook, L.: Mechanism of action of the benzodiazepines: behavioral aspect. *Federation Proceedings* 39: 3024–3031, 1980a.

Sepinwall, J., and Cook, L.: Relationship of gamma-aminobutyric acid (GABA) to antianxiety effects of benzodiazepines. *Brain Research Bulletin* 5: 839–848, 1980b.

Shader, R. I.: *Manual of Psychiatric Therapeutics.* Boston: Little, Brown, 1975.

Sherman, A. D., Allers, G. L., Petty, F., and Henn, F. A.: A neuropharmacologically relevant animal model of depression. *Neuropharmacology* 18: 891–893, 1979.

Sidman, M.: *Tactics of Scientific Research.* New York: Basic Books, 1960.

Siegel, S.: Tolerance to the hyperthermic effect of morphine in the rat is a learned response. *Journal of Comparative and Physiological Psychology* 92: 1137–1149, 1978a.

Siegel, S.: A pavlovian conditioning analysis of morphine tolerance. In Krasnegor, N. A. (ed.): *Behavioral Tolerance: Research and Treatment Implications (NIDA Research Monograph 18).* Washington DC: U.S. Department of Health, Education and Welfare, Public Health Service, National Institute of Drug Abuse, 1978b.

Skinner, B. F.: The steep and thorny way to a science of behavior. *American Psychologist* 30: 42–49, 1975.

Smith, D. F.: *Lithium and Animal Behavior,* vol. 1. Montreal: Eden, 1977.

Solomon, R. L., and Corbit, J. D.: An opponent-process theory of motivation: I. Temporal dynamics of affect. *Psychological Review* 81: 119–145, 1974.

Spitzer, R. L., Skodol, A. E., Gibbon, M., and Williams, J. B. W.: *DSM-III Case Book.* Washington DC: American Psychiatric Association, 1981.

Squires, R. F.: Monoamine oxidase inhibitors: animal pharmacology. In Iversen, L. L., Iversen, S. D., and Snyder, S. H. (eds.): *Handbook of Psychopharmacology,* vol. 14. New York: Plenum Press, 1978.

Stein, L.: Habituation and stimulus novelty: a model based on classical conditioning. *Psychological Review* 73: 352–356, 1966.

Stein, L., Belluzzi, J. D., and Wise, C. D.: Benzodiazepines: behavioral and neurochemical mechanisms. *American Journal of Psychiatry* 134: 665–669, 1977.

Stolerman, I. P., Fink, R., and Jarvik, M. E.: Acute and chronic tolerance to nicotine measured by activity in rats. *Psychopharmacologia (Berlin)* 30: 329–342, 1973.

Sulser, F.: Tricyclic antidepressants: animal pharmacology (biochemical and metabolic aspects). In Iversen, L. L., Iversen, S. D., and Snyder, S. H. (eds.): *Handbook of Psychopharmacology,* vol. 14. New York: Plenum Press, 1978.

Tallarida, R. J., and Jacob, L. S.: *The Dose–Response Relation in Pharmacology.* New York: Springer-Verlag, 1979.

Tang, M., and Falk, J. L.: Behavioral and pharmacological components of phenobarbital tolerance. In Krasnegor, N. A. (ed.). *Behavioral Tolerance: Research and Treatment Implications (NIDA Research Monograph 18).* Washington DC: U.S. Department of Health, Education and Welfare, Public Health Service, National Institute of Drug Abuse, 1978.

Tessel, R. E., and Woods, J. H.: Fenfluramine and N-ethyl amphetamine: comparison of the reinforcing and rate-decreasing actions in the rhesus monkey. *Psychopharmacologia (Berlin)* 43: 239–244, 1975.

van Abeelen, J. H. F.: Genotype and the cholinergic control of exploratory behaviour in mice. In van Abeelen, J. H. F. (ed.): *The Genetics of Behaviour.* New York: American Elsevier, 1974.

van Kammen, D. P.: The dopamine hypothesis of schizophrenia revisited. *Psychoneuroendocrinology* 4: 37–46, 1979.

Verhave, T., Owen, J. E., Jr., and Robbins, E. B.: The effect of morphine sulfate on avoidance and escape behavior. *Journal of Pharmacology and Experimental Therapeutics* 125: 248–251, 1959.

Vogel, R. A., Frye, G. D., Wilson, J. H., Kuhn, C. M., et al.: Attenuation of the effects of punishment by ethanol: comparisons with chlordiazepoxide. *Psychopharmacology* 71: 123–129, 1980.

Vogel-Sprott, M.: Alcohol effects on human behaviour under reward and punishment. *Psychopharmacologia (Berlin)* 11: 337–344, 1967.

Wallach, M. B., and Hedley, L. R.: The effects of antihistamines in a modified behavioral despair test. *Communications in Psychopharmacology* 3: 35–39, 1979.

Wenger, G. R.: Some quantitative behavioral pharmacology in the mouse. In Thompson, T., and Dews, P. B. (eds.): *Advances in Behavioral Pharmacology,* vol. 2. New York: Academic Press, 1979.

Wise, C. D., Berger, B. D., and Stein, L.: Benzodiazepines: anxiety-reducing activity by reduction of serotonin turnover in the brain. *Science* 177: 180–183, 1972.

Wise, R. A., and Dawson, V.: Diazepam-induced eating and lever pressing for food in sated rats. *Journal of Comparative and Physiological Psychology* 86: 930–941, 1974.

Woods, J. H.: Behavioral pharmacology of drug self-administration. In Lipton, M. A., DiMascio, A., and Killam, K. F. (eds.): *Psychopharmacology: A Generation of Progress.* New York: Raven Press, 1978.

Wyatt, R. J.: Biochemistry and schizophrenia (part IV), the neuroleptics—their mechanism of action: a review of the biochemical literature. *Psychopharmacology Bulletin* 12: 5–50, 1976.

Zbinden, G., and Randall, L. O.: Pharmacology of benzodiazepines: laboratory and clinical correlations. *Advances in Pharmacology* 5: 213–91, 1967.

Index